Group Process and Structure in Psychosocial Occupational Therapy

Group Process and Structure in Psychosocial Occupational Therapy

Diane Gibson
Editor

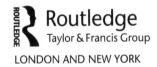

Routledge
Taylor & Francis Group

LONDON AND NEW YORK

First Published 1988 by The Haworth Press, Inc.
Published 2013 by Routledge
711 Third Avenue, New York, NY 10017 USA
2 Park Square, Milton Park, Abingdon, Oxon OX14 4RN

Routledge is an imprint of the Taylor & Francis Group, an informabusiness

Group Process and Structure in Psychosocial Occupational Therapy has also been published as *Occupational Therapy in Mental Health*, Volume 8, Number 3, 1988.

LIBRARY OF CONGRESS
Library of Congress Cataloging-in-Publication-Data

Group process and structure in psychosocial occupational therapy / Diane Gibson, editor,
    p. cm.
    "Group process and structure in psychosocial occupational therapy has also been published as Occupational therapy in mental health, volume 8, number 3, 1988" —T.p. verso.
    Includes bibliographical references.
    ISBN 0-86656-829-8
    1. Occupational therapy. 2. Group psychotherapy. I. Gibson, Diane.
RC487.G76 1988
616.89'1652--dcl9
    88-15325
    CIP

ISBN 978-1-315-80409-5 (eISBN)

Group Process and Structure in Psychosocial Occupational Therapy

CONTENTS

ABOUT THE EDITOR

Diane Gibson, MS, OTR, is Director of Activity Therapy at The Sheppard and Enoch Pratt Hospital in Baltimore, Maryland, where her responsibilities include directing activity therapy treatment programs for approximately 350 hospitalized psychiatric patients of varying ages and diagnoses. She is also a senior faculty member at the Education Center, The Sheppard and Enoch Pratt Hospital. In addition to being the author of numerous publications in the occupational therapy field and a frequent lecturer on stress and management issues, she is the editor of *Occupational Therapy in Mental Health.*

Foreword

This book, *Group Process and Structure in Psychosocial Occupational Therapy*, is dedicated to assisting occupational therapy practitioners and students in understanding current theory and techniques in group treatment. New therapists tend to join the work force armed with sufficient information about diagnoses and task analysis, yet lacking in both knowledge and skills necessary to conduct groups. Effective group leadership need not, indeed, should not be left to the initiative and ingenuity of the therapist.

Structural elements such as goals, norms, group size, physical environment and instructions can be varied depending on the purpose, needs and functional level of the clients. Being able to guide and control process elements, such as spontaneous feedback, supports clients and helps build a cohesive, safe group. Articles by Howe and Schwartzberg and by Stein trace these important concepts which are elucidated by examples and protocols.

Several articles by McDermott, by Cole and Greene, and by Weaver study the differential benefits of activity based vs. verbally based groups on varying group interaction patterns and diagnoses. Outcomes described validate the efficacy of activity in promoting social interaction and community living skills. An interesting article by Hardison and Llorens traces the use of a craft group in the treatment of delinquent girls. Occupational therapists who have suffered from being unable to defend the therapeutic use of activity groups will take heart upon reading research which affirms their basic tenets.

The last three articles by Love, by Probst and Howe, and by McLean describe fascinating new group techniques which include a social skills game, a mime group, and the use of robots. These innovative techniques demonstrate how creative content can effectively combine structure and process in group treatment.

Diane Gibson
Editor

Structure and Process in Designing a Functional Group

Margot C. Howe, EdD, OTR, FAOTA
Sharan L. Schwartzberg, EdD, OTR, FAOTA

SUMMARY. An understanding of the relationship between group structure and process is necessary to ensure the maximal therapeutic benefits of group treatment. This also applies to the planning or design stage of a group. This article discusses the relation between structure and process in the context of a functional group model and addresses issues that the group leader needs to consider in planning and running a group. A group Protocol is presented to assist in this task.

The recognition of the benefits from group work in occupational therapy is nowhere more apparent than in the area of mental health. Groups are universally used for occupational therapy in mental health settings, according to Duncombe and Howe (1985), and these groups are usually activity or task groups where the goal of the group is to accomplish a task or activity. While there are many definitions of a group, Mosey's (1973) definition is appropriate: "A group is an aggregate of people who share a common purpose which can be attained only by group members interacting and working together" (p. 45). By definition then, a group has a purpose or goal, as well as a structure; namely, people interacting and working together. It is the component of group structure that will be ad-

Margot C. Howe is Professor of Occupational Therapy at Tufts University-Boston School of Occupational Therapy, Medford, MA 02155.

Sharan L. Schwartzberg is Associate Professor of Occupational Therapy and Chairwoman at Tufts University-Boston School of Occupational Therapy, Medford, MA 02155.

1

dressed in this paper; how group structure relates to process in facilitating or hindering the achievement of group goals.

All groups have structure. Group structure can be defined as the group form, the combination of mutually connected and dependent parts of a group (Howe, 1968). Group structure is composed of the organization and procedures of the group, those factors which influence the capacity of the group to reach its goals. For instance, when comparing a group that conducts its business through parliamentary procedures with a group that makes decisions in an informal manner, it is easy to see that the groups exhibit different structures. In the first group, all communication between members is channeled through the chairperson and decisions are made by majority vote. In the second group, members can communicate directly with each other without the intervention of the leader; communication can be more direct and spontaneous, and while decisions may be less orderly and more time-consuming, the results may in some cases give members greater satisfaction.

Two other traits common to all groups are process and content. The term process refers to the ways in which the work of the group is done and in the manner in which things are said. This includes how members are relating to one another in the group, who talks to whom, how decisions are made, and how group tasks are accomplished. The term content refers to what is said and discussed during the group session. Both process and content occur in every group, be it an informal gathering of friends or a formal meeting.

Group structure is formed by a number of factors, such as the nature of the goals of the group, the pattern of leadership-membership interaction, the size of the group and the composition of its members, the history of the group, and the group setting or climate. Every group exists as an individual entity and is unlike any other group as it is composed of various combinations of characteristics that make up its structure, process and content. In planning a group, therapists need to consider which of these factors can be changed and which are fixed and unalterable since the structure will influence the group process.

To clarify the relationship of structure to process we will specifically address the initial planning stages of a group using the functional group model presented by Howe and Schwartzberg (1986).

The group goals defined by this model are "adaptation and occupation (or action) and its four different forms: purposeful action, self-initiated action, spontaneous or here-and-now action, and group-centered action" (p. 95). The role of the therapist or leader in the planning phase of the group is of critical importance to the group's ultimate success. Here, the leader must establish the need for the group, determine group goals and procedures, develop a group plan, select the group members and structure the group and its activities. The leader will need to continually reassess the plan and make changes as the group evolves.

The leader needs to know how to use group structure to enhance the group process. To accomplish this result within the functional group model, the following factors should be considered in planning, running, and reviewing the group: (1) maximum involvement through group-centered action, (2) a maximum sense of individual and group identity, (3) a "flow" experience, (4) spontaneous involvement of members, and (5) member support and feedback. These five major categories should be reviewed individually in terms of the parameters to be considered by the leader or co-leaders. It is suggested that the Group Session Plan Protocol (see Figure 1) be used to organize and formulate the clinical reasoning process for group interventions.

MAXIMAL INVOLVEMENT THROUGH GROUP-CENTERED ACTION

Maximum involvement of members can be achieved by orienting the group to the design, explaining the procedures, setting up the task, and then planning a follow-up discussion. Obviously the leader needs to consider the members' level of functioning in planning how to present the group's design to the members. This is best thought out in advance of actually attempting to involve the group members. The cognitive level and socio-emotional maturity of the members are also important variables to consider. For example, it is wise to present only a few steps of an activity at a time if the group members have short attention spans, difficulty concentrating or are disoriented. In addition, the type of member activity involvement should be carefully graded to ensure a successful group experience.

Figure 1

Group Session Plan Protocol

A. Name of Group_____

   Date _____

B. Specific goals for the group session

C. Specific goals for group members if different from above, and goals
   for each group member

D. Description of and rationale for methods and   procedures

E. Description of and rationale for leadership role

F. Describe necessary preparations

G. List materal and equipment needed

H. Time and sequence outline for sessions, including what you will do
   and say as leader, and what the group will do; consider both content
   and process.

I. Other information pertinent to this specific session: For example--
   will there be any new members, co-leaders, or guests; is there an
   unusual tone on the unit or special event that is about to occur or
   just occurred for the individual member or group?

From: Howe, M.C., & Schwartzberg, S.L. (1986). A functional approach
to group work in occupational therapy. Philadelphia: J.B. Lippincott,
p. 142.

MAXIMUM SENSE OF INDIVIDUAL
AND GROUP IDENTITY

When a safe environment is created and members feel in control
of the group's process, content and progress, a sense of group identity can be achieved. In groups where there is a highly changing
membership, such as in an open group, the leader usually needs to

be the one to maintain structure for member involvement. The use of assigned membership roles and tasks is one way of ensuring individual identity as well as participation in the group process. Leaders may also choose to label groups with names that reinforce the group identity such as "the men's group," "the exercise group" or "the Lucky 13 Club." This may be particularly important when members' ego boundaries or self-identities are unclear. Naming may also increase pride in the group, such as with a group composed of adolescents.

A FLOW EXPERIENCE

The concept of a flow experience according to Csikszentmihalyi (1975) is: "The state of flow is felt when opportunities for action are in balance with the actor's skills . . ." (p. 49). In order to achieve a flow experience, the group leader must look at the expectations that the group will have for the members, so that the group does not demand performance that is above the members' capabilities. At the same time, the leader avoids having members perform at a level below their performance capabilities. The design should ultimately incorporate an activity process that all members are capable of accomplishing, so that they feel they are in control of the situation. A co-leader relationship can also demonstrate a means by which people can work cooperatively on a task to achieve mutually desired satisfaction. The range of activities common in occupational therapy groups makes it easy to adapt the group's materials, processes and products to assure a flow experience. Where member capabilities are widely divergent it may be necessary to split the group into two groups of more homogeneous membership.

SPONTANEOUS INVOLVEMENT

Here-and-now action is essential to achieving spontaneous involvement. The leader attempts to be a model for the group members and to structure a supportive environment for experiential learning in the present. A group member who is relatively unskilled in interpersonal relations may learn interpersonal skills by observing the leader model. The structure of the group may also facilitate member involvement through helping to establish the legitimate group norms, value, and limits of behavior. The leader is viewed as the central person or spokesperson of the group and his or her overt behavior strengthens the norms and values of the group. Effective leaders spend time in their groups explaining to the members why they do what they do and why they structure the group in a particular way. They also share with the members their perceptions of how members interact with each other in specific instances. Leaders also create spontaneous involvement by giving members feedback in an empathetic manner and by being receptive to member feedback.

The activities are structured so that the action is in the present and will require spontaneous involvement and response. Nevertheless, in formulating a session plan, the leader still identifies a time sequence for the meeting's activities. It is surprising to new group leaders that spontaneity is more likely to occur when activities are planned therapeutic interventions. Matching meaningful tasks with member interests and abilities, involving group members in the group plans, and avoiding criticism in the group, all contribute to a climate of spontaneity. To achieve spontaneous involvement the leader must also put energy into creating a feeling of safety in the group, especially in protecting new members in the initial group meetings.

MEMBER SUPPORT AND FEEDBACK

In the planning stage, the leader needs to include group experiences in which member support and feedback occur. This frequently entails leader demonstrations as to how support and feedback are given. Leaders must also encourage group members to support one another and to build this into the group's activity structure and process. The plan should include opportunities to teach ways of giving and receiving feedback. This may include learning principles such as avoiding criticizing another group member or blaming them for the group's failure.

In planning for a closed group that will meet over a period of time, changes in structure must be considered as the group progresses through various stages. Even in an open group or short-term group, individual sessions follow a developmental pattern. Each session is a microcosm of a sequence of meetings of long-term groups, the periods being shorter and more superficial than in ongoing groups. The leader must plan with these changes in mind.

During the early group sessions, as members seek to find acceptable group behavior, they look to the leader for direction and structure as well as approval. The beginning leader may be undecided as to how much structure to provide. Yalom (1983) writes:

> Although patients desire and require considerable structuring by the therapist, excessive structure may retard their therapeutic growth. If the leader does everything for patients, they will do little for themselves. Thus, in the early stages of therapy, structure provides reassurance to the frightened and confused patient; but persistent and rigid structure, over the long run, can infantalize the patient and delay assumption of autonomy. (p. 123)

The leader may use the natural structure of the group or the structure of the task to provide a safe environment for members who are new to the group. This safe climate may give way for greater risk-taking as the group progresses. The leader needs to remember that group development doesn't necessarily progress in a smooth course. The group may need to return to a safer climate from time to time.

As control can be a major problem for some people, the leader will want to keep the need for control in mind in planning the group sessions. Again both the structure of the group and of the task can be effectively used to determine the desired process. For instance, if a group of adolescents has trouble accepting adult leadership, the leader can select a task with inherent limits and controls which in turn provides members with a sense of being in control themselves. An activity that includes such factors as steps that are repeated, activities that are known to the members, objects that are familiar, and materials that are easily controlled could be appropriately selected.

The purpose of this paper was to identify how the design stage of a group can be used to develop insight in determining the balance between structure and process in occupational therapy group work.

Five factors were offered for consideration in planning and reviewing group interventions:

1. Maximum involvement through group-centered action;
2. Maximum sense of individual and group identity;
3. A "flow" experience;
4. Spontaneous involvement; and
5. Member support and feedback.

Finally it is important to remember that groups require ongoing evaluation (Howe & Schwartzberg, 1986). Individual session plans need to be continuously adapted as the needs of members change and the group naturally evolves in its unique ways.

REFERENCES

Csikszentmihalyi, M. (1975). *Beyond boredom and anxiety: The experience of play in work and games*. San Francisco: Jossey-Bass.

Duncombe, L.W., & Howe, M.C. (1985). Group work in occupational therapy: A survey of practice. *American Journal of Occupational Therapy*, 39(3): 163-170.

Howe, M. (1968). A Review of Selected Professional Literature Describing Four Youth Groups to Determine Structure with References to Psychiatric Occupational Therapy. Unpublished Master's Thesis. San Jose State University.

Howe, M.C., & Schwartzberg, S.L. (1986). *A functional approach to group work in occupational therapy*. Philadelphia: J.B. Lippincott.

Mosey, A.C. (1973). *Activities therapy*. New York: Raven Press.

Yalom, I.D. (1983). *Inpatient group psychotherapy*. New York: Basic Books.

Applying the Group Process
to Psychiatric Occupational Therapy
Part 1:
Historical and Current Use

Franklin Stein, PhD, OTR, FAOTA
Beverlea K. Tallant, MA, OT(C)

SUMMARY. The authors trace the current use of group activities in occupational therapy from an historical perspective. A pilot study of thirty-four psychiatric treatment programs located in Wisconsin, Quebec, and Alberta are described. The five most frequent groups used in these facilities include: social skills training, independent living skills, leisure time activities, stress management and exercise. The results are compared to a previous study by Duncombe and Howe, 1985.

Group therapies were first developed historically as a means to encourage patients to gain insight into their illnesses and to foster self-expression. In the present practice of group therapy a diversity of theories and methods have emerged that can be readily applied by the psychiatric occupational therapist. In this paper the authors trace the history of group therapy in psychiatry and in occupational therapy. The authors describe the most widely used group therapy methods and the current use of groups by psychiatric occupational therapists.

The authors raise the following questions in this paper:

Franklin Stein, Director, Occupational Therapy Program, University of Wisconsin-Milwaukee.

Beverlea K. Tallant, Occupational Therapy Program, School of Physical and Occupational Therapy, McGill University, Montreal, Canada.

9

What are the historical precursors to the development of group treatment?

Who are the major group theorists?

What are the current frames of references and methods used in group occupational therapy?

How are groups currently being used in psychiatric occupational therapy?

HISTORICAL DEVELOPMENT
OF GROUP THERAPY

Group therapy, a method of working with disabled patients, began during the 1920s. It coincided with the psychoanalytic movements of Freud, Adler and Jung and the introduction of psychotherapy as a treatment method. In the initial practice of group therapy, clinicians used lectures and discussion methods to encourage patients to gain insight into the psychodynamics of their illnesses and to foster mutual understanding from the members of the group. For example: J. H. Pratt (1922), working with tuberculosis patients in a Boston hospital, used educational lectures to inspire patients and to increase their motivation to regain their health. Lecture methods which encouraged patient discussion were also used by early practitioners of group therapy. Lazell (1921) lectured to schizophrenic patients as a method of increasing self-awareness. Alfred Adler (1930) used group methods in working with emotionally disturbed children and their parents as a way of providing mutual problem solving approaches, when he worked in child guidance clinics in Vienna. J. L. Moreno (1946) initiated psychodrama as a method to help psychiatric patients re-experience and act out traumatic events in their lives. Moreno experimented actively with psychotherapy during the 1920s in Vienna and later introduced these techniques into the United States. Moreno was the first group psychotherapist to develop a formal methodology in using group processes with psychiatric patients. He emphasized the importance of catharsis, i.e., the expression of emotional feelings that have been repressed, in the treatment of schizophrenic patients. Another important contributor to the development of group methods in treatment was S. L. Slavson (1964) a social worker who worked with emotionally disturbed children during the 1930s in New York City. Slavson used arts and crafts activities and play media to help the child to express conflicts and emotions without the interference of the group therapist. Slavson felt this approach was most useful with repressed and withdrawn children who needed to release their feelings without parental and adult censure and disapproval. Group therapy methods were used sparingly in mental hospitals before the 1930s. L. C. Marsh (1935) a minister and psychiatrist, used discussion groups in class settings for examining everyday issues such as the family, child development, job problems and social interactions. In these groups patients were encouraged to support each other. Paul Schilder (1939), a psychoanalytically trained psychiatrist, used group therapy methods to foster individual insight and self-confidence with others while he was at Bellevue Hospital in New York City in the 1930s.

After the Second World War group therapy was increasingly used in psychiatric hospitals and clinics throughout the United States. During this time group methods developed from theoretical frameworks such as nondirective therapy (Rogers, 1968), behavior therapy (Wolpe, 1969), transactional analysis (Berne, 1966), gestalt therapy (Perls, Hefferline, & Goodman, 1951) and the therapeutic community (Jones, 1953).

Activity Group Therapy

This method, developed initially by Slavson (1964), has been incorporated into group occupational therapy and can be applied most effectively with hyperactive children who must develop the inner controls for self-regulation (Cermak, Stein, & Abelson, 1973).

In Slavson's approach the children are encouraged to act out conflicts and emotions without the intervention of the therapist. The group meets for approximately an hour and a half using creative media such as finger paints, watercolors, modeling clay or paper crafts. The therapist establishes an emotional climate of unconditional acceptance and trust. The group is composed of about eight children of the same age or sex. An emotional balance in the group is fostered by the therapist by placing very aggressive children in with passively withdrawn children. At the end of the activity session, the therapist and children share a neutral activity such as having a "snack."

Slavson's model is very much influenced by psychoanalytic theory and it is primarily designed to provide emotionally disturbed children a permissive environment in which to encourage unrestrained expression of feelings (Rosenbaum & Snadowsky, 1976).

Directive-Didactic Approach

This group experience relies upon the therapist to guide discussions and activities of specific areas of importance in patient treatment and rehabilitation. The therapist uses educational methods, such as lectures, film, slides, video-tapes and seminar discussions. Content areas include prevocational exploration, family dynamics, understanding yourself, sexual adjustment, health maintenance, nutrition, exercise or other areas of interest and importance. In this approach the therapist designs the group experience as similar to a college course syllabus. The behavioral objectives of the group are defined, the specific content areas are described, and audiovisual programs are listed (Klapman, 1963).

Client-Centered Rogerian Group

The core of Rogerian therapy is the concept that man has the potential for self-actualization. In Client-Centered approaches the therapist emphasizes the healthy aspect of the individual rather than the disability or illness. The therapist is a democratic treatment agent in the group fostering an atmosphere of positive self-regard. The therapist attempts to facilitate personal growth in the individual by eliciting statements describing the client. One of the most important concepts in this approach is self-ideal congruence. In this concept the therapist works toward helping the client develop self-awareness and to compare how the client perceives his/her self with how the client would ideally like to be. Progress is assessed by how the client narrows the perceptual discrepancy between present self and ideal self (Meador, 1975).

T-Group

The T-Group methodology developed in 1947. The sponsor of this methodology was the National Training Laboratory for Group Development which held the first formal program for sensitivity training (Golembiewski & Blumberg, 1977). The T-Group has three distinguishing features, i.e., it is a learning laboratory simulating a miniature society, it focuses on learning how to learn, and there is strong emphasis on the here and now in relation to ideas, feelings and reactions. The prime task of the trainer (group leader) is to establish a psychologically safe atmosphere that facilitates learning. The task of the group members is to examine their behavior in interpersonal relationships. For example, if an individual obtains insight into his behavioral characteristics, then it is felt that the person will be able to express himself consistent with his inner feelings and ideas. The main goals of T-Groups are to improve an individual's quality of cognition, clarify his identity, increase his self-esteem, self-acceptance, and acceptance of others. The philosophy of a T-Group is similar to Roger's theory, however, the methodologies are much more formal. For example, the leader of a group undergoes a formal period of observation before becoming certified. In addition to Roger's theory, T-Groups rely heavily on the theories of Lewin (1951), a psychologist who analyzed social forces in the environment that affect individual behavior.

Psychodrama

The application of a creative art form as a therapeutic methodology is consistent with occupational therapy. Moreno, a psychiatrist living in Vienna during the early nineteen-hundreds, established the theatre of spontaneity (Moreno, 1946). "The objective of psychodrama was from its inception to construct a therapeutic setting that uses life as a model, to integrate into the setting all the modalities of living — beginning with the universals of time, space, reality and the cosmos — and moving down to all the details and nuances of life" (Moreno, 1983, p. 158). The important components of psychodrama are the *stage* where the life dramas are re-enacted; the *protagonist* who is the center of the drama; the *auxiliary egos* are the other individuals, e.g., patients or staff, who act out the protagonist's family or significant individuals in the protagonist's life; the *director* or therapist, who guides the drama and is critically aware of the significance of what is happening in the patient's behavior; and the *audience* who can take an active part in the action by reacting, responding and evaluating the action. The audience can also serve in the role of consensual validator relating objectively to the protagonist's working through of emotional issues. Psychodrama has been used with all types of diagnostic categories in psychiatric hospitals and in community mental health facilities. It is a formal method that has been adapted and modified by psychiatric occupational therapists to accommodate for special needs. Role playing, simulated life dramas and behavioral rehearsal are techniques inspired from psychodrama.

Transactional Analysis (TA)

Eric Berne, a psychiatrist and psychoanalyst, developed the technique of Transactional Analysis during the 1950s. Transactional Analysis is a method of therapy based on examining the interpersonal exchanges that occur in social encounters. Berne identifies basically three roles that individuals assume in social interactions, i.e., the child, parent and adult. These three ego states are similar to but not the same as Freud's concept of id, superego and ego (Berne, 1966). The child ego state is characterized by unrestrained emotional expression, play-like behavior and a need to be nurtured and protected. The parent ego state is characterized by a judgmental and critical attitude toward others. The parent is ready to overprotect others and to make decisions in an authoritarian manner. The adult ego state is the healthiest and most democratic transaction. The adult shares decisions with others and is a responsible self-accepting individual. Every individual assumes these three ego states, during his or her daily interactions with others. Some environments, such as a spectator at a sports event, encourage child-like behavior, while leading discussions may elicit an adult ego state and disciplining a child will elicit a parent ego state. In group therapy situations using transactional analysis, the therapist can act as a parent interpreting behavior and providing insight for the patient. The occupational therapist in working with patients can also function as a parent authority figure, or adult sharing responsibility or as a child participating with the patients in group activities.

Gestalt Therapy

This humanistic approach to treatment was created primarily from the work of Fredrick Perls (1969). Applying the concepts of Gestalt Psychology to treatment, Perls emphasized the wholeness of the individual and the awareness of the here and now. The gestalt therapist tries to help the individual discover who he or she is and to fully experience these feelings. Individual growth is equated with the individual becoming more aware of his/her senses. The individual is taught not to analyze his feelings but to describe them. Gestalt therapists use sensory-awareness exercises, role playing, and experimental encounters that help the individual to be in contact with the immediate environment. Individuals are taught how to be in touch with their feelings and to understand how feelings are generated. The therapist creates an open, genuine environment for the patient in which to experiment with interactions and feelings without the fear of making mistakes in the encounters. The therapist also is encouraged to express feelings in a genuine, authentic manner.

Behavioral Group Therapy

Learning principles and techniques such as behavioral group contracts, positive reinforcement, time-out, token economy, shaping, modelling, behavior rehearsal, cognitive restructuring, relaxation and imagery have been utilized in group therapy (Feldman & Wodarski, 1975). The behavioral group therapy approach has been found particularly effective for phobics who fear social evaluative situations such as public-speaking (Paul & Shannon, 1966), for underassertive physically disabled university students (Morgan & Leung, 1980), for individuals who lack social interaction skills, and for acting-out aggressive behaviors seen in emotionally disturbed adolescents (Feldman & Wodarski, 1975).

Generally the client receives individual treatment first and then is placed in group therapy for a more advanced level of treatment (Wolpe, 1982). The advantage of the group setting is that it gives the client the opportunity to practice new behaviors in a more "in vivo" situation.

USE OF GROUP ACTIVITIES IN PSYCHIATRIC OCCUPATIONAL THERAPY

In the 1800s the use of activity with psychiatric patients in a small group setting was introduced in France (Leuret, 1948), the United States of America (U.S.A.) (Meyer, 1977), and Canada (Driver, 1968). These early activities consisted of gardening, laundry, and construction of hospital buildings (Driver, 1968). By the early 1900s these work activities were supplemented with recreational, craft and social group activities which became known as "occupational therapy classes" (Driver, 1968). Meyer (1977) felt the primary benefits of these groups were to control patient "excitements" or mischievous behaviour, decrease boredom and increase socialization.

Activity Groups

Eleanor Clarke Slagle (Hopkins & Smith, 1978) developed a scheme of resocializing and reintegrating patients starting with individual crafts in a group setting (basketry) leading up to work preparation groups for hospital jobs such as cooking, gardening, farming, etc. From the early 1930s through the forties, several occupational therapists (Howe & Schwartzberg, 1986) recognized the socialization value of group activity and had the patients work together on a common task or project such as quilt-making, games, or work.

Self-Awareness Groups

The influence of the Fidlers (Fidler, G. & Fidler, J., 1954) and the Azimas (Azima, H. & Azima, F., 1959a) on psychiatric occupational therapy was considerable. As proponents of the analytic frame of reference, they introduced the concept of object-relationships, the dynamic use of objects on a one to one basis and the utilization of psychotherapeutic techniques (Fidler & Fine, 1962) in occupational therapy. It was not long before they saw the potential of the group to "facilitate treatment" (Fidler, G. & Fidler, J., 1954).

At that time, the Fidlers (Fidler, G. & Fidler, J., 1954) had patients work in a group setting primarily as a means to increase social awareness, responsibility and cooperation and to develop a sense of belonging. The group setting was used to meet general rather than specific goals for the patient. Later, they used group projects or competitive games to foster group cohesion. This approach is still used with specific populations, such as mothers with depression, to provide a supportive, educative and participatory setting which will help maintain the individual in the community and prevent rehospitalization (Campbell, 1975; Gracegirdle, 1982).

The Azimas, however, used unstructured creative activities with a group of patients for the purpose of group psychotherapy (Azima, Cramer-Azima, & Wittkower, 1957). The group participated in free creative and free association activities using pencil and paper, crayons or plasticine as media. The objectives of the group were to work through defenses, drives, conflicts, transference, and to help the patient gain insight into their feelings and behaviour. In a later paper (Azima, H. & Azima, F., 1959b), they discussed the importance of the created object as an essential catalyst in the group process.

Currently, occupational therapists continue to use the creative media of art, music, poetry, clay, and role-playing to help patients to project, confront, and gain insight into their inner conflicts and feelings (Blair, 1974; Monroe & Herron, 1980; Lindsay, 1983).

Reality-Oriented Groups

In 1959, the American Occupational Therapy Association (AOTA) (West, 1959) advocated the therapeutic use of groups and group activities in psychiatric occupational therapy. It recognized three main types of groups, that is, adult education, social, and group psychotherapy. The proceedings of the Allenberry Conference presented the objectives for each type and highly recommended that occupational therapists be trained in group process and group leadership.

Group therapy mushroomed in the sixties due to the impact of

Maxwell Jones' concept of the therapeutic community (1953). The use of a group as a primary therapeutic entity became accepted (Reed & Sanderson, 1980). In occupational therapy the purpose of group activities was to encourage ego growth, communication skills, reality-testing and functional independence (Fidler, G. & Fidler, J., 1963; German, 1964). Group activities usually consisted of a didactic lecture component, task or practicum component and discussion. For example, an Activities of Daily Living Discussion Group (German, 1964) for females would consist of hearing and discussing specific topics (Art appreciation, Children and child care, Extracurricular activities), group readings on a topic, verbal or visual demonstrations, and community outings in conjunction with the topic.

Role-Oriented Groups

Mary Reilly (1974) emphasized the importance of roles in life such as worker, parent, friend, spouse. This led occupational therapists to develop group activities to help patients develop the skills necessary for healthy functioning within a given role. Work training groups (Furner, 1978) focused on the theory and practice of developing work skills by taking patients through a 10 week series of topics and tasks solely related to work. The results were that 21 of the treated group (N = 31) were able to be discharged from hospital with nine finding employment, eight attending a community work assessment agency, and four attending a day hospital.

Developmental Groups

The developmental frame of reference was described by Anne Cronin-Mosey (1970) as a viable treatment approach in occupational therapy for psychiatric patients. Within this frame of reference, the development of "Group Interaction Skills" was viewed as an essential element of maturation. Mosey (1970) delineated the ages and sequence in which these skills would normally develop. The skills ranged from parallel group activity (18 months-2 years), similar to the parallel play of children, to mature group participation at 15 to 18 years of age. The mature group member is able to take on several group membership roles and attain satisfaction both from the task and group participation.

An initial assessment is made to determine the patient's dysfunction in group interaction skills. The patient is placed in group activities which match his current developmental level. The patient is then slowly exposed to and "matured" through higher level groups so that they can acquire the appropriate group interaction skills for their chronological age (Broekema, Dany, & Schloemer, 1975).

Behavioral Groups

Principles of learning (Mosey, 1970) have influenced the type and format of group activities used in psychiatric occupational therapy. Behavioral techniques, such as the systematic use of positive and negative reinforcement, extinction, shaping, modelling, behavioral rehearsal and feedback, have been used with both chronic and acute patients.

Basic skills of daily living such as eye contact, grooming, cooking and work habits have been taught, shaped and reinforced by the use of a token economy system (Kaye, Mackie, & Hitzing, 1970; Schell & Giles, 1985). Social skills training has been used to help adolescents control delinquent behaviours (Schell & Giles, 1985), to develop listening and communication skills in chronic patients (Hewitt, Wishart, & Lambert, 1981; Drouet, 1986), and to help patients overcome acute anxiety in social or friendship situations (Davis & Keene, 1983). Appropriate assertiveness has been developed in anxious, underassertive clients through a combination of lectures on assertion and assertive techniques, role-playing, homework, and feedback from the group (Wojnar-Horton & Jansons, 1982).

Human Occupation Groups

The model of human occupation (Kielhofner, 1980) views the human being as an integrated system made up of subsystems which are concerned with performance, habituation and volition. In this theory, the higher levels govern the lower ones, so that one's values or interests could overcome environmental obstacles. Conversely, dysfunction at the lower level (performance) could constrain the higher ones. For example, a newly blinded artist may no longer be able to paint and, therefore, must seek other media or means of creative expression.

Clients are assessed on each subsystem and treatment is directed at those deficits. If an individual has good performance and habit skills but no desire to use them they might participate in a group activity which is directed toward values clarification. However, if a client has performance deficits, treatment might focus on basic skills such as perceptual-motor, communication and interaction skills through a highly structured, directive group process (Kaplan, 1986).

Cognitive Dysfunction Groups

Recent advances in the neuroscientific understanding of brain function enables the role that cognitive dysfunction plays in functional behavior to be better understood. Claudia Allen (1985) proposes that careful assessment of a patient's cognitive disabilities permits placement in activities which have been accurately matched to their level of function. She delineated six levels of cognitive dysfunction. Level 1 means that the client is conscious, reflexes are working, however, attention and awareness are seriously impaired. Level 6, the top level, is considered to be normal, involves planned actions and the ability to use symbolic cues.

Earhart (1985) describes nine occupational therapy groups which may be used to treat the six levels of cognitive dysfunction. The groups range from simple movement (Level 2), grooming and basic crafts (Levels 3 and 4), basic educational skills (Level 4) to ones which involve higher levels of organization such as cooking and work evaluation (Levels 5 and 6). She discusses the ideal number and type of patients as well as specific activities for each group level. Guidelines are provided for the occupational therapist in terms of setting up the group environment, equipment and manner of instruction. Each group description includes examples of the observed cognitive disabilities for specific psychiatric conditions.

A quick look at the eighties indicates that the use of group activities in psychiatric occupational therapy is an integral part of any program (Duncombe & Howe, 1985). The purpose of group activity has changed markedly from the early 1900s (Meyer, 1977) when it was primarily used to increase socialization or control behavior. Modern day practice, with its advantages of technology (Holm, 1983), is one in which the type of group activity and selection of patients are carefully planned. The purpose of each group activity is determined by the particular theoretical frame of reference, the type of group process desired, and the specific treatment goals of the group members.

CURRENT USE OF GROUPS IN PSYCHIATRIC OCCUPATIONAL THERAPY

In the winter of 1986, a pilot survey of thirty-four psychiatric programs was carried out to determine the present practice of psychiatric occupational therapy (Stein & Brintnell, 1986). Data were obtained from either an on-site interview (62%) or mail survey (38%). Of the thirty-four psychiatric facilities surveyed, eighteen (53%) were in-patient units in a General Hospital, six (17%) were Day Treatment Centers, four (15%) were county or State Mental Hospitals, four (12%) were Extended Care Facilities or Nursing Homes and one (3%) was a Veterans Administration Hospital. The major DSM-III diagnosis treated in these facilities, ranked in order according to frequency, included: schizophrenia disorders, affective disorders, organic mental disorders, substance abuse, personality disorders and anxiety disorders. As part of the survey, questions were developed to identify the type of treatment groups that are currently part of the occupational therapy program. Table 1 describes the results of the survey. It is interesting to note that the majority of the facilities used treatment groups that are based on the behavioral model of teaching functional abilities such as social skills, independent living skills, cognitive training and prevocational training. The groups are also goal directed toward improving coping mechanisms such as stress management, values clarification and assertiveness training. The other three groups; i.e., exercise, leisure time activities, and expressive/creative are related to a holistic approach to the patient.

In a related question, the investigator examined the frequency of activity modalities used in occupational therapy. The specific types

Table 1

Percent and Ranking of Occupational Therapy

Treatment Groups in 34* Psychiatric Facilities

Treatment Group	Percent Present in all 34 Facilities	Frequency of Ranked First
Social Skills Training	94%	14
Independent Living Skills	91%	7
Leisure Time Activities	88%	1
Stress Management	79%	2
Exercise Group	71%	1
Values Clarification	65%	2
Assertiveness Training	59%	0
Prevocational Training	47%	1
Expressive/Creative	23%	0
Cognitive Training	12%	0

----

* Facilities were surveyed in Wisconsin, Montreal, Quebec and Alberta, Canada

of activities were identified by the respondent (see Table 2). These activities are considered with the types of treatment groups reported. For example independent living skills, cooking, and arts and crafts are used in almost every facility. These modalities are the bases for group treatment. Relaxation therapy, role playing, creative arts, assembly tasks, and table games are also frequently used in psychiatric occupational therapy. The treatment groups and modalities can be interpreted as a definition of the role function of the psychiatric occupational therapist. We can infer from these preliminary data, that occupational therapists in psychiatry use group treatment techniques and modalities to increase social skills, independent living functions, leisure and creative activities, stress management-relaxation therapy, and prevocational abilities.

In a prior study, Duncombe and Howe (1985) surveyed 120 therapists employed in general hospitals, rehabilitation centers, psychi-

Table 2

Frequency and Percentage of Activity Modalities used in
Psychiatric Occupational Therapy Program

n = 34

Activity Modality	Yes	Percent	No	Percent
Cooking	33	97	1	3
Independent Living Skills	32	94	2	6
Arts and Crafts	32	94	2	6
Relaxation Therapy	30	88	4	12
Assembly Tasks	30	88	4	12
Table Games	27	79	7	21
Role Playing	26	76	8	24
Creative Arts	25	75	9	26
Community Field Trips	22	65	12	35
Sports	20	59	14	41
Films, Music Appreciation	18	53	16	47
Prevocational Tasks	16	47	18	53
Educational Courses	10	29	24	71
Microcomputers	1	3	33	97

atric facilities, nursing homes and community programs. Of the 120 responding therapists, 72 or 55% used groups in treatment. The 72 who used groups characterized 54% of the groups as activity groups and 24% as verbal groups. Based on their data, ten categories of groups were identified, i.e., exercise, cooking, activities of daily living, arts and crafts, self-expression, feeling-oriented, reality-oriented, sensory-motor and sensory integration, and educational groups. The descriptions of these groups are below:

Exercise: Patients performed physical exercise to increase coordination, mobility and strength.
Cooking: Combined tasks of meal planning, shopping, cooking and eating.

Activities of Daily Living: Issues focussed upon included transportation, grooming, time and money management and use of leisure.

Arts and Crafts: Included ceramics, leather, copper tooling, wood working, macrame, rug hooking, needlework, weaving and art.

Verbal Groups

Self-Expression: Used art, group collage, role-playing or self-awareness activities.

Feeling-Oriented Discussion: Used role playing, poetry, fantasy and description of current life situations.

Reality-Oriented Discussion: Topics included current events, discharge planning, program planning, goals for treatment, use of time and daily patient concerns.

Sensori-motor and Sensory Integration Groups: Included gross and fine motor activities, as well as sensory activities for tactile, taste and vestibular stimulation, and were targeted for children.

Education Groups: These groups were organized to provide information to patients about medications, joint protection for arthritis and family planning.

In comparing the results from the two studies it is important to note that the first survey (Stein & Brintnell, 1986) was limited to psychiatric facilities only while the second study (Duncombe & Howe, 1985) included mail questionnaire data from both psychiatric and non-psychiatric programs. Duncombe and Howe also distinguished between verbal versus activity groups. This is a dubious distinction that does not accurately describe the group phenomena. Activity groups to some extent are verbal in that the activities are explained and the patients have the opportunity to discuss their reactions to the activity. Groups that use only verbal interactions excluding role playing, collage, art, music, dance, and so on should be categorized as psychotherapy or group treatment. Most occupational therapists who categorize their groups as verbal usually incorporate some type of media into their sessions. A more accurate analysis of groups would include the frame of reference, e.g., psychoanalytic, behavioral, gestalt, client-centered; the goals of the group, e.g., increase social skills, improve independent living skills, increase stress management; and the structural aspects of the group such as number of patients, sessions per week and the length of each session.

It is evident from these two pilot studies that further research is needed to examine objectively in a more precise manner the nature of groups used in psychiatric occupational therapy.

CONCLUSION

In this paper, the authors have reviewed the development of group therapy. The use of group activities in psychiatric occupational therapy has been traced historically to the present. The different types of groups used have been discussed within a chronological context.

The results of a recent survey conducted on the use of groups in 34 psychiatric occupational therapy facilities have been presented. A comparison has been made with another survey on the use of groups in occupational therapy in general. In each case, it is evident that group activities are widely used as treatment by occupational therapists.

In conclusion, it is clear that occupational therapists must have a thorough knowledge of the group process as well as the essential skills to be an effective group leader in working with psychiatric patients.

REFERENCES

Adler, A. (1930). *Guiding the child*. New York: Greenberg.

Allen, C. (1985). *Occupational therapy for psychiatric diseases: Measurement and management of cognitive disabilities*. Boston: Little, Brown and Company.

Azima, H., Cramer-Azima, F., & Wittkower, E.G. (1957). Analytic group art therapy. *The International Journal of Group Psychotherapy, 7*, 243-260.

Azima, H., & Azima, F. (1959a). Outline of a dynamic theory of occupational therapy. *American Journal of Occupational Therapy, 13*, 215-221.

Azima, H., & Azima, F. (1959b). Projective group therapy. *International Journal of Group Psychotherapy, 9*, 176-183.

Berne, E. (1966). *Principles of group treatment*. New York: Oxford University Press.

Blair, A. (1974). Projective techniques: Their application within a group psychotherapy situation. *Proceedings 6th International Congress, World Federation of Occupational Therapy*, Vancouver, 365-379.

Broekema, M., Danz, K., & Schloemer, C. (1975). Occupational Therapy in a community after care program. *American Journal of Occupational Therapy, 29*, (1), 22-27.

Campbell, D. (1975). Project Alternative, a therapeutic social group. *Canadian Journal of Occupational Therapy, 42*, 145-149.

Cermak, S., Stein, F. & Abelson, C. (1973). Hyperactive children and a group activity therapy model. *American Journal of Occupational Therapy, 27*, 311-315.

Davis, S., & Keene, N. (1983). Making social skills work with outpatients. *Occupational Therapy, 46*, 257-259.

Driver, M. (1968). A philosophic view of the history of occupational therapy in Canada. *Canadian Journal of Occupational Therapy, 35*, 53-60.

Drouet, V. (1986). Individual behavioural programme planning with long-stay schizophrenic patients. Part 2: Social skills training. *Occupational Therapy, 49*, 229-231.

Duncombe, L., & Howe, M. (1985). Group work in occupational therapy: A survey of practice. *American Journal of Occupational Therapy, 39*, 163-170.

Earhart, C. (1985). 10. Occupational therapy groups. In C. Allen, *Occupational therapy for psychiatric diseases: Measurement and management of cognitive disabilities*. Boston: Little, Brown and Company.

Feldman, R., & Wodarski, J. (1975). *Contemporary approaches to group therapy*. London: Jossey-Bass Publishers.

Fidler, G., & Fidler, J. (1954). *Introduction to psychiatric occupational therapy*. New York: The Macmillan Company.

Fidler, G., & Fine, S. (1962). The occupational therapist and psychotherapy. *Transitional programs in psychiatric occupational therapy*. Study Course Manual III. International congress of the World Federation of Occupational Therapists.

Fidler, G., & Fidler, J. (1963). *A communication process in psychiatry – occupational therapy*. New York: The Macmillan Company.

Furner, L. (1978). Work training groups. *Occupational Therapy, 41*, 232-233.

German, S. (1964). A group approach to rehabilitation occupational therapy in a psychiatric setting. *American Journal of Occupational Therapy, 18*, 209-214.

Golembiewski, R., & Blumberg, A. (Eds.) (1977). *Sensitivity training and the laboratory approach* (3rd ed.). Itasca, IL: Peacock Publishers.

Gracegirdle, H. (1982). A group for depressed mothers and their children. *Occupational Therapy, 45*, 20-21.

Hewitt, K., Wishart, C., & Lambert, R. (1981). Social skills training with chronic psychiatric patients. *Occupational Therapy, 44*, 284-285.

Holm, M. (1983). Video as a medium in occupational therapy. *American Journal of Occupational Therapy, 37*, 531-534.

Hopkins, H., & Smith, H. (1978). *Willard and Spackman occupational therapy/ Fifth edition*. Philadelphia: J.B. Lippincott Company.

Howe, M., & Schwartzberg, S. (1986). *A functional approach to group work in occupational therapy*. Philadelphia: J.B. Lippincott Company.

Jones, M. (1953). *The therapeutic community: A new treatment method in psychiatry*. New York: Basic Books.

Kaplan, K. (1986). The Directive Group: Short-term treatment for psychiatric patients with a minimal level of functioning. *American Journal of Occupational Therapy, 40*, 474-481.

Kaye, J., Mackie, V., & Hitzing, E. (1970). Contingency management in a workshop setting: Innovation in occupational therapy. *American Journal of Occupational Therapy, 34*, 572-581.

Kielhofner, G. (1980). A model of human occupation. Part 1: Conceptual framework and content. *American Journal of Occupational Therapy, 34*, 572-581.

Klapman, J. (1963). The case for didactic group psychotherapy. In M. Rosenbaum and M. Berger (Eds.) *Group Psychotherapy and Group Functions*. New York: Basic Books.

Lazell, E.W. (1921). The group treatment of dementia praecox. *Psychoanalytic Review, 8*, 168-179.

Leuret, F. (1948). On the moral treatment in insanity. In S. Licht (Ed. and Trans.) *Occupational Therapy Source Book*. Baltimore: Williams & Wilkins Company (Article originally written in 1840).

Lewin, K. (1951). *Field Theory in Social Science*. New York: Harper.

Lindsay, W. (1983). The role of the occupational therapist treatment of alcoholism. *American Journal of Occupational Therapy, 37*(1), 36-43.

Marsh, L.C. (1935). Group therapy and the psychiatric clinic. *Journal of Nervous and Mental Disorders, 32*, 381-392.

Meador, B.D. (1975). Client-centered group therapy. In G. Gazda, (Ed.) *Basic Approaches to Group Psychotherapy and Group Counseling* (2nd ed.). Springfield, IL: Charles C Thomas.

Meyer, A. (1977). The philosophy of occupational therapy. *American Journal of Occupational Therapy, 31*, 639-642.

Monroe, C., & Herron, S. (1980). Projective art used as an integral part of an intensive group therapy experience. *Occupational Therapy, 43*, 21-24.

Moreno, J.L. (1946). *Psychodrama*. New York: Beacon House.

Moreno, Z. (1983). Psychodrama. In H. Kaplan, and B. Saddock (Eds.), *Comprehensive Group Psychotherapy*. Baltimore: Williams and Wilkins.

Morgan, B., & Leung, P. (1980). Effects of assertion training on acceptance of disease by physically disabled university students. *Journal of Counselling Psychology, 27*, 209-212.

Mosey, A. (1973). *Activities therapy*. New York: Raven Press.

Mosey, A. (1970). *Three frames of references for mental health*. New Jersey: Charles B. Slack, Inc.

Paul, G., & Shannon, D. (1966). Treatment of anxiety through systematic desensitization in therapy groups. *Journal of Abnormal Psychology, 71*, 124.

Perls, F., Hefferline, R., & Goodman, P. (1951). *Gestalt therapy excitement and growth in the human potential*. New York: Julian Press.

Perls, F. (1969). *Gestalt therapy verbatim*. New York: Bantam.

Pratt, J.H. (1922). The principles of class treatment and their application to various chronic diseases. *Hospital School Service, 6,* 401.

Reed, K., & Sanderson, S. (1980). *Concepts of occupational therapy*. Baltimore: The Williams and Wilkins Company.

Reilly, M. (1974). *Play as exploratory learning*. Beverly Hills: Sage Publications, Inc.

Rogers, C. (1968). *The process of the basic encounter group*. La Jolla, CA: Western Behavioral Sciences Institute.

Rosenbaum, M., & Snadowsky, A. (1976). *The intensive group experience: A guide to therapy, sensitivity encounter, self-awareness group, human relations training and communes*. New York: The Free Press.

Schell, D., & Giles, G. (1985). Behaviour modification with disturbed adolescents: The role of the occupational therapist. *Occupational Therapy, 48,* 172-178.

Schilder, P. (1939). Results and problems of group psychotherapy in severe neurosis. *Mental Hygiene, 23,* 87-98.

Slavson, S.R. (1964). *Textbook in analytic group psychotherapy*. New York: International Universities Press.

Stein, F. & Brintnell, E.S. (1986). Survey of thirty-four occupational therapy programs located in psychiatric facilities in Wisconsin, Alberta and Quebec. Unpublished Study.

West, W. (1959). *Changing concepts and practices in psychiatric occupational therapy*. New York: American Occupational Therapy Association.

Wojnar-Horton, S., & Jansons, L. (1982). Assertion training in a community health centre. *8th International Congress, World Federation of Occupational Therapists*, Hamburg, Germany, 991-998.

Wolpe, J. (1969). *The practice of psychotherapy*. New York: Pergamon Press.

Wolpe, J. (1982). *The practice of behaviour therapy*. New York: Pergamon Press.

Applying the Group Process to Psychiatric Occupational Therapy Part 2: A Model for a Therapeutic Group in Psychiatric Occupational Therapy

Franklin Stein, PhD, OTR, FAOTA
Beverlea K. Tallant, MA, OT(C)

SUMMARY. Extensive literature on group treatment and a model for initiating a therapeutic group in psychiatric occupational therapy are examined by the authors. In this review a structural analysis of the group is discussed, i.e., group goals, cohesiveness, therapeutic contracts, selection of patients, leadership styles, time and place considerations, group models, therapeutic media and the evaluation of a group's effectiveness. Examples of reality orientation, values clarification and the soap opera as a dynamic group approach are described.

INTRODUCTION

Occupational therapists traditionally work with psychiatric patients in groups. The interrelationships and personal interactions in groups have an excellent potential for therapeutic change. The group functioning at an optimum level represents a microcosm of each individual's social world. The communications, interactions, and emotional expressions that occur in the group are used by the group leader and members of the group to effect positive growth

---

Franklin Stein, Director, Occupational Therapy Program, University of Wisconsin-Milwaukee.

Beverlea K. Tallant, Occupational Therapy Program, School of Physical and Occupational Therapy, McGill University, Montreal, Canada.

and change. If the group is to be successful in producing therapeutic results and patient recovery then the occupational therapist must plan carefully how it will be used.

The purposes of this paper are to examine the critical factors and issues in forming a therapeutic group and to present a model for initiating a therapeutic group in occupational therapy.

A MODEL FOR A THERAPEUTIC GROUP IN PSYCHIATRIC OCCUPATIONAL THERAPY

The group situation lends itself to a structural analysis that can guide the occupational therapist to use the group process most effectively. The structural analysis of groups includes such questions as: How does one initiate a therapeutic group? How often should the group meet? What are the most appropriate therapeutic activities of groups? What are the goals? What is the leadership style of the occupational therapist in the group? How can the occupational therapist increase the cohesiveness of the group? How does one enhance the effectiveness of group occupational therapy? If group treatment is to be used effectively with psychiatric patients, the therapist must be aware of these factors. In Table 1, a sequential analysis of the factors that are important in initiating a group are presented.

1. Group Goals Are Established

Yalom (1975) identified a number of factors that contribute to the curative factors in group therapy. These factors listed below are also relevant to occupational therapy.

Instillation of hope in the client or patient. The therapist must convey the positive benefits to be derived from group therapy. In a way it is using a positive placebo effect. As Yalom points out, the success of self-help groups such as Alcoholics Anonymous and Recovery, Inc., are based on the strong conviction and faith that the method works. Group occupational therapy is an effective method to help the client develop self-esteem, interpersonal skills, consensual validation and social competencies. In many instances, it is "the treatment of choice for a widening range of patients with highly diverse problems" (Kaplan & Saddock, 1983).

TABLE 1

SEQUENTIAL ANALYSIS OF A THERAPEUTIC GROUP IN OCCUPATIONAL THERAPY

1	2	3	4
Group Goals are Established	Structure for Established Goals Identified	Administrative Contract Established	Patients Selected
examples: -understanding self -interpersonal learning -prevocational exploration -instillation of hope -sharing of feelings	-time period -number of patients -length of sessions -cohesiveness -environment where group will meet	-approval of group members consistent with group goals	-considers variables such as diagnosis, sex, age, treatment goals and patient motivation

5	6	7	8
Therapeutic Leadership Styles Recognized	Group Methodology Identified	Media Selected	Group(s) Effectiveness Evaluated
democratic (therapist shares leadership with members) -laissez-faire (free expression) -authoritarian (therapist controlled)	-lecture discussions -free expression -simulate interpersonal situations -individual life assessments -task-oriented -sensory awareness -reality-orientation	-audio-visual -arts and craft activities -prevocational activities -value clarification exercises -music -dance -poetry -drama -cooking, etc.	-psychometrics -self-reports -family and staff evaluation

Universality or sharing of experiences. The group experience conveys to the patient that his or her experiences are not unique. Many times it is comforting to the patient to know that other individuals with severe depression, delusions, anxieties, and phobias have improved. The patient can come to realize that he/she is not alone. The patient also begins to disclose feelings about which he/she may have previously felt ashamed or guilty. The ability to share feelings with a group of individuals who are willing to listen without judging one's behavior is therapeutic. The group members can be supportive, confrontive, empathic and understanding. The individual member can gain valuable feedback regarding how others see him/her and can gain self-insight through the therapeutic group process (Azima & Azima, 1959).

Imparting of information. The group is an excellent vehicle for imparting information to the client using methods of lecture, seminar-discussions and role playing. Mini courses targeted for vulnerable groups such as widows, alcoholics, drug addicts, single parents, in community settings as well as for psychiatric in-patients, can be designed for a specified period of time such as once a week for four months (Gracegirdle, 1982; Lindsay, 1983). Guest speakers, films or field trips can be incorporated into the mini course organized by the occupational therapist (German, 1964). For example, mini courses can involve such topics as Re-entering the Job Market; Stress Management; Holistic Health; Accident Prevention in the Home; Parent Effectiveness and Interpersonal Skills. The occupational therapist can skillfully establish therapeutic groups that are content oriented and create a supportive climate that allows for individual development. Frequently, the occupational therapist may work as a co-therapist with other members of the mental health team such as the psychologist, psychiatrist, nurse or social worker.

Altruism, as Yalom (1975) defines it, in the group is observed when members are "helpful to one another. . . . They offer support, reassurance, suggestions, insight and share similar problems with one another." The occupational therapist can create a climate of altruism in the workshop or clinic while patients are working on projects. It is not unusual for the occupational therapist to encourage patients to help each other on craft or group projects. This mutual assistance is beneficial to both the "altruist" and the patient receiving the "altruism." For example, in producing a ward newspaper, patients can separate the individual tasks of writing poetry and/or feature stories, typing, designing, collating, stapling, etc., based on each one's skills and capacities. The occupational therapist serves as a catalyst in these relationships helping the patients to help each other. In this way, the therapist encourages the development of mutually dependent relationships which lead to the success of the project. The therapist positively reinforces the mutual working together of the group members. The occupational therapist can also create situations in which patients can work through potential personality conflicts by demonstrating mutual assistance.

Simulate family structure. The group process can be used effectively to work through family problems (Anthony, 1971). Patients with prior difficulties with parents, siblings and significant others many times project their feelings and preconceived ideas to other patients in the group. The group can be used as a laboratory in which to experiment with new interactions as well as to recreate situations to resolve "smoldering" conflicts.

Role playing, where patients act out family roles, is effective in groups. The occupational therapist as a co-leader with a psychologist or social worker in this group can incorporate group exercises and activities to stimulate group interaction.

Family drawings depicting the patient's position in relationship to other family members can be used in a group to stimulate self-awareness and insight (Burns, 1982). The group members can interpret the drawings in a climate of support and mutual understanding.

Values clarification exercises can be used to elicit the individual's personal values in relation to career goals, friends, responsibility and commitment to ideals (Corey, 1985, p. 443-445). These group exercises can aid the patient in developing a tolerance for others with different values and a respect for differences among family members.

Redevelopment of basic social skills. Hersen and Bellack (1977) define social skills as the:

> . . . ability to express both positive and negative feelings in the interpersonal context without suffering consequent loss of social reinforcement. Such skill is demonstrated in a large variety of interpersonal contexts . . . and it involves the coordinated delivery of appropriate verbal and nonverbal responses.

In addition, the socially skilled individual is attuned to the realities of the situation and is aware when he is likely to be reinforced for his efforts. . . . (p. 512)

The group process can be used to improve social skills training by re-enacting interpersonal situations. The occupational therapist can prepare an environment for simulating listening skills, verbal responses, non-verbal communication, initiating conversation, and maintaining a relationship. Group exercises can be incorporated into the group process such as using videotapes of role playing and re-enactments of social interactions (Wachtel, 1983).

2. Structure of the Group Identified

Before initiating a therapeutic group, the occupational therapist must consider the following questions and issues:

a. What are my qualifications and experiences in leading a therapeutic group? Do I need specialized skills and advanced training in group therapy methods before I can be effective?

b. Will supervision be available to me during the group process so that I can prevent personality conflicts with patients and be maximally effective in interpersonal growth?

c. Should I lead the group myself or with a co-leader such as another occupational therapist, social worker, psychologist, psychiatrist or nurse?

d. What patients should be selected for the group? Should the group be homogeneous regarding age, sex, diagnostic category or degree of chronicity?

e. How large should the group be? Should the group be voluntary or required as part of the treatment program?

f. Should any interested patients be allowed to enter the group at any time (open-ended) or should membership be controlled by screening criteria (closed)?

g. How long should the group meet and over what period of time? Should the group be an open ended group where patients enter and leave informally or should the group meet for a specified period of time, e.g., three months for an hour and a half, twice a week?

h. What activities will be incorporated into the group? Will arts and crafts media, group games, interpersonal exercises, or audiovisual equipment be incorporated into the group?

i. What is the most effective environment for the group to use? Is the space adequate for meeting the needs of the group and the activities planned?

j. How should the patient be initiated into the group? Should the occupational therapist meet individually with potential group members before meeting with the group as a whole?

k. How should the occupational therapist document the content of group discussions and member interactions? Should audiovisual equipment be used to record the group process?

l. How should the progress of individual members of the group be communicated to the mental health team?

m. How should the group exercises be incorporated with other therapeutic activities?

n. How can the occupational therapist evaluate the cohesiveness of the group and the individual progress of patients in the group?

Group Cohesiveness

The structure of the group should facilitate group cohesiveness if it is planned well. Group cohesiveness is defined (Cartwright & Zander, 1968) as the resultant of all the forces acting on all members to remain in the group. In other words, group cohesiveness is a positive factor in the group that is related to an individual's desire to participate and share experiences with other people. It is a "sine qua non" for therapeutic effectiveness. It provides the basis for social interactions and interpersonal learning. It also is an important factor in fostering attendance of individual members in the group and their willingness to share in group decisions.

On the other hand, groups that fail to establish cohesiveness are less likely to succeed (Bednar & Kaul, 1978). Attendance will decline, patients will become apathetic and the group will dissolve itself. Group cohesiveness is an important indicator for the occupational therapist when evaluating the group's effectiveness. If the individual finds personal satisfaction and looks forward to group participation, then the occupational therapist can conclude that the group process is facilitating cohesiveness. Before the group can become effective with individual patients, there must be a climate of trust and mutual understanding established where the individual feels emotionally secure and can reveal his/her conflicts and interpersonal problems. The point when group cohesiveness is reached, is the point when the group begins to function as a positive environment for personal growth.

3. Administrative and Therapeutic Contracts

Are the group's goals consistent with the goals of the treatment facility? For example, if an occupational therapist is interested in setting up a group for prevocational exploration, do the other professional staff members understand the importance of the group? Do they see its functions and goals as consistent with the overall treatment goals of the facility? The administrator of the treatment facility usually must make a decision when the group's operations involve space needs, budget implications and the patient's family approval. The administrative contract exists between the occupational therapist initiating the group, the clinical director of the program, or the administrator of the facility, depending upon whoever is most appropriate in granting administrative approval. The contract usually is in the form of a memo requesting approval by the occupational therapist for initiating a new group. In the memo the therapist states the number of patients to be in the group, where the group will meet, the time for the group, the total number of group sessions, the overall goals and the space and equipment requirements of the group.

The therapist's contract is the agreement between the therapist and patient regarding the responsibilities and functions of each in the group. In a therapeutic group it is expected that the members of the group are selected individually based on their potential to benefit from the group experiences. In the therapeutic contract, which can either be verbal or written, the therapist states the overall goals for the group, the time commitment, the type of activities to be used in the group and the responsibilities of the patient, which implies an agreement to take an active part in the group. It is important to raise the expectations of hope for the patient in the group, otherwise the patient may be ambivalent about becoming involved. The success of the group will depend, in the final analysis, on the activity and motivation of the patients. The therapeutic contract is a method to increase the motivation of the patient to use the group experience most effectively.

4. Selection of Patients

In the selection of patients for a group, the therapist considers the size of the group, the composition of group members and screening criteria for group inclusion (Yalom, 1975).

Most researchers and clinicians working with groups consider that the size of a group should range from as few as five members to not more than about fifteen. The ideal group size for therapy is considered to be between six and eight members (Battegay, 1974). The size of a group should facilitate each member to active participation. If the group is too large, individuals are fearful of disclosing their inner-most feelings. On the other hand, if the group is too small, individuals may lose interest and become bored with each other. A group of eight individuals seems to be a good balance as the individual can establish interpersonal relationships with each member of the group while enough diversity of experiences is generated to maintain interest in the group. If one considers that a group usually meets for less than ninety minutes, it is highly probable that in a group of ten individuals there will be less than ten minutes of time for each member to actively participate.

In considering the composition of the group the occupational therapist must determine if the group will be homogeneous in regard to sex, age, marital status, education, and socioeconomic status, for example, as in groups such as Alcoholics Anonymous and single parent support groups. Yalom (1975) recommends that groups be composed with "heterogeneity for conflict areas and homogeneity for ego strength." In a way, Yalom is recommending that individuals with a variety of diagnoses be mixed together in groups to create a type of suspense and curiosity about the other people in the group. However, the group members should be equal in their abilities to protect their egos and in their abilities to accept criticism and to cope with the psychodynamics revealed in the group.

The occupational therapist must also be cognizant of members who are unable to identify with the majority in the group and, who, therefore, become isolated and cut off from the mainstream of the group.

In screening potential members for a therapeutic group, the occupational therapist must consider whether the individual will benefit from the group process. This question relates to the individuals' therapeutic goals and their compatibility with the group's goals. Not all individuals will benefit from groups and it is important for the occupational therapist to keep this in mind when selecting potential members. Will the potential member be motivated to contribute positively to the group? Will the member identify with the other group members? Is the individual able to share the attention of the therapist with other group members? The occupational therapist must settle these issues before any recommendations are made.

5. Therapeutic Leadership Styles

The role of the occupational therapist in the group is an important factor that is considered before the group meets. Should the occupational therapist assume a domineering authority role in the group or should the therapist take a less active role and serve mainly as a facilitator for the group? The literature on leadership roles in groups differentiates between democratic, laissez-faire and authoritarian leadership styles (White & Lippitt, 1968). These three styles imply levels of control by the occupational therapist in the group. In the democratic group, decisions are made by the total group and the leader is responsive to the group's desires. In the laissez-faire group, the group is essentially leaderless and decisions are made by the individual group members and accepted or rejected by others. In the authoritarian leadership, the occupational therapist plans the goals for the group and guides the group's progress. All final decisions for the group are made by the therapist.

In actual group settings, it may be useful for the occupational therapist to use all three leadership styles depending upon the goals of the group. It is also apparent that in groups where the members are unable or unwilling to make decisions, as with emotionally disturbed children or chronic schizophrenic in-patients, the therapist may have to assume an authoritarian role. On the other hand, certain groups such as T-Groups are structured to be democratic. The amount of control that the therapist assumes in the group will have an important effect in the success of the group (Cartwright & Zander, 1968).

6. Group Methodology

Occupational therapy group methods can be divided into five major areas:

   a. *Didactic Group.* In this group the occupational therapist uses lectures, audiovisual aids and other learning techniques to develop social skills, individual competencies or general knowledge. For example, areas of adult education can be used to stimulate interest in the patient and to facilitate social interaction. Poetry reading groups, art and music appreciation groups, film groups and other similar groups can be organized around patient interests. In these groups the therapist acts as a catalyst and therapeutic leader to stimulate the patient's desire to learn, and develop vocational and leisure time activities (Rance & Price, 1973). (See Appendix A — "Reality Orientation.")

   b. *Projective Group.* Drawing, sculpture, puppetry, collage, drama and other creative media are used to help the patient communicate feelings and ideas to others (Blair, 1974; Horowitz, 1971; Monroe & Herron, 1980; Shuman, Marcus & Nesse, 1973; Zink, 1975). The therapist creates a climate of free expression to help each individual to feel comfortable in sharing his/her creative expressions with others. The therapist can stimulate the group by suggesting that the group members, for example, express through finger painting their most happy moment in life, or recreate an event that had an important impact on their life. Background music can be used to generate an emotion. After the members complete their creative expression, each member is given the opportunity to describe his/her production. The other members of the group freely interact during this process. (See Appendix B—"Personal Coat of Arms.")

c. *Simulated Group*. In a prevocational simulated group, issues are centered around career selection, job satisfaction, and strategies for looking for a job. These areas are explored in the group through role playing, value clarification exercises and individual life assessments (Desmond & Seligman, 1977).

Versluys (1980) presents a model for the use of role-focused groups to help disabled individuals to continue responsibility for role tasks that are temporarily lost because of hospitalization. In this simulated group, the patients are provided the opportunities to "test their ability to deal with problems of living, decision making and risk taking . . ." (p. 611). Specific role-focused group models are further elaborated. For example, a *homemaking group* with emphasis on child care, cooking, architectural and interior design; *role maintenance group* with emphasis on community and social interactions with agencies and friends; *social skills development group* that explores leisure time activities such as chess, bowling, and musical activities which can be shared by participants; *sensitivity training group* that emphasizes interpersonal relationships (see Appendix C—"The Soap Opera") and transitional groups that are designed to help the patient bridge the gap between hospital and community.

d. *Task-Oriented Group*. In this type of group, the main energy is devoted to reaching goals, finding solutions to a problem, or building a product (Kaplan & Saddock, 1983). A cooking group is an example of a task-oriented group that is used frequently by occupational therapists. In this group, patients work cooperatively on various aspects of the task such as planning a menu, shopping, preparing the food, serving and dining (Broekema, Danz & Schloemer, 1975). Each aspect of the task-oriented group is focused on the finished product. The tasks in the group necessitate cooperative behavior and create cohesiveness among the group members. Other task-oriented groups include redecorating an area, planning and carrying out a social event, fund raising for a social cause, creating and producing a film (Holm, 1983), and discussing a political issue with the goal of writing a group position paper.

e. *Sensory Awareness Group.* In this group the occupational therapist structures the group experience to help the patient to become aware of his bodily sensations and to facilitate bodily relaxation. Progressive relaxation exercises can be incorporated into a group to encourage a sharing of feelings and reactions to learning how to relax. Jacobson (1958) introduced relaxation training as a behavioral approach to reducing tension, anxiety and hypertension. Jacobson proposed that individuals learn to relax by becoming aware of their muscle sensations by recognizing the difference between muscle tenseness and muscle relaxation in the major joints of their bodies. This information is later used by patients to learn how to relax and to incorporate this exercise into their everyday life.

An unorthodox approach to sensory awareness exercises was developed by Feldenkrais (1972). In this approach the individual becomes newly acquainted with his body by flexing and extending his joints, positioning his body parts and moving his body through unfamiliar sequences. Nonhabitual and habitual movements are juxtaposed. Under the guidance of the therapist, the individual stretches muscles, swings his body, and feels his body balancing and adjusting to change. The sensory awareness exercises elicit reactions and interchanges between the group members.

7. Selection of Therapeutic Media

A therapeutic medium is defined by Wilkinson and Heater (1979) as "any activity that is utilized to achieve specific goals for remediation, restoration, growth, and development or prevention . . ." (p. 1). Therapeutic media are utilized in groups to facilitate group goals. In Table 2, activities are identified that can be used effectively with specified populations. Some activities have intrinsic characteristics that are more appropriate for meeting the specific needs of the patient. The selection of the activity depends to a large degree on the nature of the group members, i.e., their age, education, dysfunction, motivation, setting and ego strength. The selec-

Table 2

Relationship Between Therapeutic Media and Group Goals

Therapeutic Media	General Advantages	Goal Applications
Audio-visual, e.g. television, playback simulations	Allows for individual to evaluate performance skills objectively	Facilitate social competencies and interpersonal skills
Arts and Crafts e.g. water color, finger painting	Permit individual creation of unique products	Self awareness, release of feelings
Values Clarification Exercises, e.g., Personal Coat of Arms	Provide opportunities to make personal de- cisions	Increase self- understanding
Prevocational Activities	Stress individual's abilities	Provide for explor- ation of vocational interests and work skills on job.

tion of the activity should be tied to problem solving issues in the patient's life (Earhart, 1985). The therapist has a wide range of creative and structured activities available that allow the individual to express his/her feelings such as art, movement, poetry and music. Still other activities facilitate decision-making and problem solving such as value clarification exercises and prevocational exploration.

Activities such as cooking, audiovisual playback and psychodrama can be used to facilitate social interaction. Activities are vehicles for the occupational therapist to achieve therapeutic goals. The occupational therapy group is different, then, from traditional group therapy led by psychologists and psychiatrists in that the occupational therapist incorporates activity media, group games, non-verbal exercises and role-playing in the group process. The variety of media that are available to the occupational therapist can be selected carefully to facilitate group interest.

8. Evaluation of a Group's Effectiveness

An effective group enables individual members to improve. How can the occupational therapist objectively evaluate a group's effectiveness? The first step in evaluating effectiveness is to operationally define the goals of the group. Examples of group goals and related measures are listed in Table 3.

In measuring progress of specific outcome variables in the group, the occupational therapist can merely count the number of behavioral responses expressed by a group member, have the member keep a diary of personal reactions, observe and document verbal and non-verbal communications, design tailor-made evaluations or surveys of group behavior, or use standardized personality tests. In some instances, an independent observer/leader of the group sessions has been used. The observer's assessment of a client's progress has then been compared with the self-assessment of the client (Cabral & Paton, 1975).

Mosey (1970) presents an innovative model for observing and determining a patient's level of group-interaction skills. In this evaluative model the therapist selects an activity that encourages collaborative interaction for a group of between five and seven patients. The therapist observes the patients' levels of interaction in the group and checks the appropriate description in the form shown in Table 4. This information is later used in a counseling interview between the therapist and the patient.

Technical methods to record the group process such as audio or video cassette recordings are helpful as learning experiences for the members (Holm, 1983) and also can be used in documenting be-

Table 3

Operational Goals for Group Effectiveness

Group Goals	Members/Leader Observations
a. Consistent attendance	Records Kept
b. Cohesiveness	Members expressing positive desire to be in group
c. Personal growth	Members expressing self-insights
d. Increased social-interactions	Degree of participation and interactions between members.
e. Positive effect	Emotional climate of group Supportive of group goals
f. Improved listening skills	Focused attention, able to feed back
g. Respect for others	Social interactions indicated
h. Increased self-disclosure	Quality of responses and depth of information revealed
i. Self-esteem	Personal adjectives expressed in group
j. Self-control of feelings	Emotional reactions to confrontations and implied criticism
k. Empathy	Understanding and recognition of feelings of others

havior that can later be analyzed by the therapist and/or group members.

Regardless of the method used to evaluate the effectiveness of the group process, it is important for the occupational therapist to give careful consideration to operationalizing an objective criteria for defining the group's goals.

CONCLUSION

The group process applied to psychiatric treatment comprises a variety of theories, approaches and specific methodologies derived

Table 4

Mosey's Group-Interaction Skills Survey*

Type of Group

Parallel Group
        Engages in some activity, but acts as if this is an individual
                task as opposed to a group activity.
        Aware of others in the group
        Some verbal or nonverbal interaction with others
        Appears to be relatively comfortable in this situation
Project Group
        Occasionally engages in the group activity, moving in and out
                according to his own whim
        Seeks some assistance from others
        Gives some assistance when directly asked to do so
Egocentric-Cooperative Group
        Aware of group's goal relative to the task
        Aware of group norms
        Acts as if he belongs in the group
        Willing to participate
        Meets esteem needs of others
        Able to get others to meet his esteem needs
        Recognize rights of others
Cooperative Group
        Makes own wishes, desires, and needs known
        Participates in group activity but seems concerned primarily with his
                own needs and needs of others
        Able to meet needs other than esteem needs
        Tends to be most responsive to group members who are similar to him
                in some way
Mature Group
        Responsive to all group members
        Takes a variety of task roles
        Takes a variety of social-emotional roles
        Able to share leadership
        Promotes a good balance between task accomplishment and satisfaction
                of group members' needs

---

*Mosey, A. (1970). Activities Therapy. New York: Raven Press, p. 92.
Permission granted to reprint table by Raven Press.

from Activity Group Therapy, Directive-Didactic, Client-Centered, T-Group, Psychodrama, Transactional Analysis, Gestalt Therapy, and Behavioral Group Therapy.

The occupational therapist, by adapting these theories and methods and adding that unique element of occupational therapy the analyzed task or "activity," can meet specific patient treatment goals. The occupational therapist can adapt any of these theories and methods to specific patient treatment goals. What the patient gains from these experiences will depend upon the effectiveness of the occupational therapist in establishing a cohesive group that will facilitate the group goals. The group can be structured to aid the patient to increase social interactions, enhance self-esteem, improve communication skills, develop empathy, and learn greater self-awareness. Groups commonly used by psychiatric occupational therapists are didactic, projective, simulated, task-oriented, and sensory awareness groups.

It is crucial to the success of the group process that the occupational therapist possess the personal qualities, advanced training, and leadership skills that are necessary to be an effective group therapist.

REFERENCES

Anthony, E.J. (1971). An introduction to family group therapy. In Kaplan H. and Saddock B. (Eds.), *Comprehensive Group Psychotherapy*. Baltimore: The Williams and Wilkins Co.

Azima, H. & Azima, F. (1959). Projective group therapy. *International Journal of Group Psychotherapy, 9*, 176-183.

Battegay, R. (1974). Group psychotherapy as a method of treatment in a psychiatric hospital. In S. de Schill, *The Challenge for Group Psychotherapy*. New York: Universities Press, Inc.

Bednar, R. & Kaul, T. (1978). Experiential group research: Current perspectives. In S. Garfield and A. Bergin (Eds.), *Handbook of Psychotherapy and Behavior Change* (2nd ed.). New York: John Wiley & Sons.

Blair, A. (1974). Projective techniques: Their application within a group psychotherapy situation. *Proceedings 6th International Congress, World Federation of Occupational Therapy*, Vancouver, 365-379.

Broekema, M., Danz, K., & Schloemer, C. (1975). Occupational Therapy in a community after care program. *American Journal of Occupational Therapy, 29*(1), 22-27.

Burns, R. (1982). *Self-Growth in Families: Kinetic Family Drawings (K-F-D): Research and Application*. New York: Brunner/Mazel.

Cabral, R. & Paton, A. (1975). Evaluation of group therapy: Correlations between clients and observer's assessments. *British Journal of Psychiatry, 126*, 475-477.

Cartwright, D. & Zander, A. (1968). *Group dynamics: Research and theory*. New York: Harper and Row.

Corey, G. (1985). *Theory and practice of group counseling* (2nd ed). Monterey, CA: Brooks/Role Publishing Co.

Desmond, R. & Seligman, M. (1977). Groups with occupational and vocational goals. In M. Seligman (Ed.), *Group counseling and group psychotherapy with rehabilitation clients*. Springfield, IL: Charles C Thomas.

Earhart, C. (1985). Occupational therapy groups. In C. Allen, *Occupational ther-*

apy for psychiatric diseases: Measurement and management of cognitive disabilities. Boston: Little, Brown and Company.

Falk-Kessler, J. & Froschauer, K. (1978). The soap opera: A dynamic group approach for psychiatric patients. *American Journal of Occupational Therapy, 32,* 317-319.

Feldenkrais, M. (1972). *Awareness Through Movement.* New York: Harper and Row.

German, S. (1964). A group approach to rehabilitation occupational therapy in a psychiatric setting. *American Journal of Occupational Therapy, 18,* 209-214.

Gracegirdle, H. (1982). A group for depressed mothers and their children. *Occupational Therapy, 45,* 20-21.

Hart, G. (1978). *Values clarification for counselors.* Springfield, IL: Charles C Thomas.

Hersen, M. & Bellack, A. (1977). Assessment of social skills. In A. Ciminero, D. Calhoun, and H. Adams (Eds.), *Handbook for personal assessment.* New York: John Wiley & Sons.

Holm, M. (1983). Video as a medium in occupational therapy. *American Journal of Occupational Therapy, 37,* 531-534.

Horowitz, M. (1971). The use of graphic images in psychotherapy. *American Journal of Art Therapy, 10,* 153-162.

Jacobson, E. (1958). *Progressive relaxation.* Chicago: University of Chicago Press.

Kaplan, H.I. & Saddock, B.J. (Eds.) (1983). *Comprehensive group psychotherapy* (2nd ed.). Baltimore, MD: The Williams and Wilkins Co.

Lindsay, W. (1983). The role of the occupational therapist treatment of alcoholism. *American Journal of Occupational Therapy, 37*(1), 36-43.

Monroe, C. & Herron, S. (1980). Projective art used as an integral part of an intensive group therapy experience. *Occupational Therapy, 43,* 21-24.

Mosey, A. (1970). *Activities Therapy.* New York: Raven Press.

Rance, C. & Price, A. (1973). Poetry as a group project. *American Journal of Occupational Therapy, 27*(5), 252-255.

Shuman, E., Marcus, D., & Ness, D. (1973). Puppetry and the mentally ill. *American Journal of Occupational Therapy, 27,* 484-486.

Simon, S., Howe, L., & Kirschenbaum, H. (1978). *Values clarification* (2nd ed.). New York: A. and W. Publishers.

Tess, L. (1978). Alamitos-Belmont Hospital, Reality oriented group. In F. Livingston and N. O'Sullivan (Eds.), *Occupational therapy consulting in the skilled nursing facility . . . An overview.* Los Angeles, CA: Southern California Occupational Therapy Consultants.

Versluys, H. (1980). The remediation of role disorders through focused group work. *American Journal of Occupational Therapy, 34,* 609-614.

Wachtel, A.B. (1983). Videotape and group therapy. In H. Kaplan and B. Saddock (Eds.), *Comprehensive group psychotherapy* (2nd ed.). Baltimore: Williams and Wilkins.

White, R. & Lippitt, R. (1968). Leader behavior and member reaction in three "social climates." In Cartwright, D. and Zander, A., *Group dynamics research and theory* (3rd Ed.). New York: Harper and Row.

Wilkinson, V. & Heater, S. (1979). *Therapeutic media and techniques of application: A guide for activities therapists*. New York: Van Nostrand Reinhold Co.

Yalom, I. (1975). *The theory and practice of group psychotherapy* (2nd ed.). New York: Basic Books.

Zink, T. (1975). Poetry: A therapeutic tool. *Canadian Journal of Occupational Therapy, 42,* 151-154.

APPENDIX A:
REALITY ORIENTATION

Reality orientation is a group technique that was developed by a psychiatrist, James Folsom, at the Veteran's Administration Hospital in Topeka, Kansas during the latter part of the 1950s. This method was originally intended for geriatric patients who had been hospitalized for long periods of time and had become overly dependent upon the hospital nursing staff. Institutional patterns of care created chronically dependent individuals who developed symptoms of senility and social withdrawal.

The general objectives of a reality orientation group are to:

1. Minimize confusion, disorientation, and physical regression;
2. Maintain the individual level of awareness of the environment;
3. Restore the individual's sense of reality;
4. Improve psychological functioning;
5. Maintain the individual's maximum level of independent functioning in activities of daily living.

A model for a reality orientation group that can be incorporated into a geriatric treatment program in occupational therapy is presented below based on the experiences at the Alamitos-Belmont Rehabilitation Hospital. Long Beach, California (Tess, 1978).

REALITY ORIENTATION GROUP FORMAT

Number of patients:	Five.
Number of sessions:	Group meets five times a week for a half an hour at a specific place.
Material aids:	Reality boards (made of wood with slots to display information), blackboards, bulletin boards, felt boards, mock-up clocks, name tags, calendars and large bright pictures of food or familiar objects.
Environment:	Group is seated in circle or around a table.
Introductions:	Each member of the group wears a name tag and is encouraged to make bodily contact with each other.

Activity Content.
  A. Time and place — on a board with the following information, plus use of calendar, clock, and time teaching aids
     1. Name of hospital:
     2. Day and time:
     3. Month:
     4. Year:
     5. Next meal:
     6. Next holiday:
  B. Body Awareness — may use mirror
     1. Identify, move and name body parts
     2. Right and left discrimination
     3. "Draw a Man"
  C. Tactile — identify and tell if he likes how it feels
     1. Feel objects of different textures (cotton, sandpaper, etc.)
     2. Stimulation with certain objects like paint brushes
  D. Sense of smell — identify and note similarities and differences between odors
     1. Present odors such as tobacco, perfume, lemon, vanilla, etc.
     2. Associate odors and tell group about associations, i.e., lemon smell reminds me of a lemon tree in the back yard
  E. Hearing
     1. Count how many times ball bounces
     2. Rhythm instruments
  F. Sight — colors — identify primary colors
  G. Numbers
     1. Counting
     2. Writing or copying numbers
     3. Simple math — add and subtract
     4. Money — recognizing and making change
  H. Sizes and shapes — identification, color, and comparison of sizes
  I. Emotions — pictures or drawing of facial emotions
  J. Manners — use of please, thank you, may I be excused

The session ends with group singing. The leader then announces the session is over and shakes hands with each member, while announcing the time of the next meeting.

APPENDIX B:
VALUES CLARIFICATION — PERSONAL COAT OF ARMS

Hart (1978) defines values clarification as "the learning process by which people explore and clarify their values and establish plans of action based on their increased insight and knowledge about their values" (p. vii). Values clarification exercises are incorporated in sensitivity and counseling groups to facilitate self-awareness and mutual understanding. For example, in one exercise from Simon, Howe and Kirschenbaum (1978), entitled *Personal Coat of Arms*, the individual participant in the group is asked to respond to the following questions by drawing, in the appropriate area on his coat of arms, a picture, design or symbol.

1. What do you regard as your greatest personal achievement to date?
2. What do you regard as your family's greatest achievement?
3. What is the one thing that other people can do to make you happy?
4. What do you regard as your own greatest failure to date?
5. What would you do if you had one year to live and were guaranteed success in whatever you attempted?

For the sixth question the individual uses words to answer the question: What three things would you most like to be said of you if you died today?

The group members then share their coats of arms with each other disclosing their values and belief systems. The exercise helps the group members to feel close to each other and to search their lives for meaning. The occupational therapist can devise value clarification exercises adapted to specific groups or use examples from Simon, Howe and Kirschenbaum's book (1978) that lists 79 strategies for eliciting values, beliefs, and feelings.

In values clarification exercises, the individual reveals personal opinions on controversial topics, expresses interests, discloses prejudices and sets priorities. Through these exercises, the occupational therapist can create group cohesiveness and a climate of mutual self-respect. Art media, music, movement and role-playing can be incorporated with value clarification exercises to add an action dimension.

APPENDIX C:
THE SOAP OPERA: A DYNAMIC GROUP APPROACH

Television soap operas have been used by occupational therapists to serve as a catalyst for group discussions.

This group approach advantageously uses a popular media and adapts it to stimulate discussion on interpersonal relationships. Falk-Kessler and Froschauer (1978) list three objectives for the soap opera group: *behavioral* — to increase attention and concentration in the patient and to interfere with gross psychiatric symptoms such as hallucinations and bizarre behaviors; *cognitive* — to improve memory and problem-solving ability; and *interpersonal* — to improve self-awareness, communication, social interactions, and emotional identification.

In their report of this technique, a group of 10 to 15 patients met twice a week for one hour over a period of approximately four months. The group was open to all patients and regular attendance was voluntary which resulted in continual changes in membership. The television viewing took place in a living room atmosphere where the members of the group and occupational therapist watched a soap opera. A group discussion took place immediately after the viewing. Two occupational therapists guided the discussion around the character and plot of the soap opera.

The occupational therapists incorporated the techniques of modeling behavior, role playing, and psychodrama with group discussion of the soap opera. For example, the co-leaders spontaneously interacted with each other providing a model to the members, and situations evoked by the soap opera were reenacted. The members of the group were also encouraged to problem-solve situations that presented themselves in the drama. While watching the soap opera the occupational therapists recorded situational themes and possible parallels to individual members. For the process to be successful, the occupational therapists must be familiar with the individual psychodynamics of each group member and the potential areas for interpersonal conflict. At the end of the group discussion, the occupational therapist documents group discussion themes and individual reactions and behaviors during the group process.

In summary, Falk-Kessler and Froschauer (1978) found that the television soap opera presenting themes of strained interpersonal relationships, separations, rejection and family crises, is relevant to the emotionally ill and can be used effectively as a therapeutic tool for facilitating interpersonal growth.

A Preference for Activity:
A Comparative Study
of Psychotherapy Groups
vs. Occupational Therapy Groups
for Psychotic and Borderline
Inpatients

Marilyn B. Cole, MS, OTR/L
Les R. Greene, PhD

SUMMARY. This preliminary paper reports on an ongoing investigation of the interactive effects of small group structure and level of psychopathology on self and social perceptions. Specifically, psychotic- and borderline-level patients were treated and assessed in two kinds of small therapeutic groups: comparatively unstructured psychotherapy groups and more structured task-focused occupational therapy groups.

Based on current psychodynamic formulations of psychopathology, it was hypothesized, first, that the psychotic patients would respond more favorably in the structured occupational therapy groups while the borderline patients would prefer the psychotherapy groups. The data failed to substantiate this interaction, revealing, instead, a preference for the occupational therapy groups by both psychotic- and borderline-level patients.

A second hypothesis posited that the psychotic patients, in comparison to the borderline patients, would show less differentiated

Marilyn B. Cole, Assistant Professor, Department of Occupational Therapy, Quinnipiac College, and Rehabilitation Medicine Service, West Haven VA Medical Center.

Les R. Greene, Associate Professor, Department of Psychiatry, Yale University School of Medicine, and Psychology Service, West Haven VA Medical Center.

53

reactions across the two kinds of groups. Considerable support was garnered for this prediction.

Implications of the findings for clinical practice and future research are presented. A note is offered on the challenges of integrating conceptualizations from psychoanalytic psychology and theories of occupational therapy.

While the research data to date generally points to the validity of the small group as an effective treatment context for psychiatric inpatients (cf. Yalom, 1983), the extent of its usefulness and its specific kinds of effects vary in complex ways according to the personality characteristics and type of psychopathology of its members, the personality and style of its leaders, and its defined tasks and social structure. With respect to the structure or organization of the small therapeutic group, there is considerable theoretical agreement (Kernberg, 1976; Yalom, 1983) — though little systematic empirical verification — that the degree of structuring should follow levels of psychological impairment of the group participants, with greater structure and explicitness of norms, rules and roles for more severely disturbed patients. The present study was designed to provide some preliminary data bearing on this postulated relationship between degree of psychopathology and optimal structuring of small therapeutic groups. More specifically, this investigation examined the perceptions of more (i.e., psychotic) and less (i.e., borderline) disturbed psychiatric inpatients as they participated in two kinds of small therapy groups designed to vary in degree of explicit structure, namely traditional group psychotherapy and task-oriented group occupational therapy.

FRAMES OF REFERENCE

The inpatient setting in which this study was conducted offered psychoanalytically based group psychotherapy, as recently articulated by Rice and Rutan (1987). In essence this model aims at encouraging an examination of the here-and-now relationships within the group and in the milieu as a whole and at clarifying and correcting distortions that derive from a reliance upon primitive defense mechanisms and the activation of unneutralized aggressive and libidinal drives. Other than the general expectation to focus on the immediate interpersonal relations within the group, the work is largely unscripted and undirected. Analogous to the concept of blank screen in psychoanalysis, the unstructured context is seen as promoting a group process that emanates almost exclusively from the individual and collective anxieties, needs, and wishes of the group participants.

In contrast, the task-oriented occupational therapy groups in the present clinical setting reflect a very different conceptual perspective. The occupational therapist looks at engagement in activity not only as sublimation of aggressive and libidinal drives, but also as the reflection of the individual's healthy urge toward competence (White, 1971). According to Burke (1983), "occupation [is] . . . a behavior which is motivated by an intrinsic conscious urge to be effective in the environment in order to enact a variety of individually interpreted roles that are shaped by cultural tradition and learned through the process of socialization" (p. 183). Thus, the performance of tasks by patients in the occupational therapy group setting is seen as regulated not only by internal ego states, but by external physical, social and cultural forces within the environment.

With respect to the conducting of research on therapeutic small groups, the literature has consistently stressed the importance of defining the theoretical orientation and describing the structural elements of the groups being studied. Of occupational therapy groups, Scott and Ross (1987) state that "the role of activities in shaping the therapeutic medium of groups has long been a staple of occupational therapy intervention"; they emphasize the need, however, to "elaborate on the nature of activity group process and recognize the necessity to refine a rationale relevant to the special background that occupational therapy brings to group therapy" (p. 141). By virtue of their emphasis on activity, occupational therapy groups tend to require more structure than psychotherapy groups. Fidler (1969) describes a task-oriented group as one "responsible for choosing its own common task and arriving at a consensus for procedures for accomplishing that task" (p. 45). This model, which closely resembles the type of occupational therapy group used in the present study, suggests a structure centered around a shared concrete goal, but with the freedom to choose and to explore within that structure. Group members are thus expected to make decisions and act on them and to take an active role in the accomplishment of a task. Interpersonal skills are needed in this cooperative and collaborative effort and any discussion of interpersonal difficulties has a here-and-now reality focus.

Three recent studies cited by Howe and Schwartzberg (1986) bear on the structure of the task-oriented activity group. From their comparative analysis, Schwartzberg, Howe and McDermott (1982) conclude that differences in quality and quantity of social interaction are related to differences in group structure; of the three kinds of groups studied, the most interaction occurred in their activity group. Kremer, Nelson and Duncomb (1984) found that patients attach different and specific affective meaning to different kinds of activity groups. Finally, Henry, Nelson and Duncomb (1984) found that the freedom to choose specific activities in occupational therapy groups significantly affects feelings of personal potency. Taken together, these studies support the idea that the structuring of the activity group has a significant influence upon the group members, in their social behaviors, their perceptions and affective reactions.

LITERATURE REVIEW

Research relevant to the present investigation can be classified into three categories: (1) studies of the effectiveness of therapeutic groups for psychotic patients, (2) studies on group-based treatment for borderline patients, and (3) studies on the effects of group structure. Unfortunately, only a few articles were found that simultaneously involve two or three of these areas.

Group Treatment for Psychotic Patients

Numerous scientific reports on the use of group therapy for psychotic-level patients, particularly schizophrenics, have been published, especially in the years immediately following deinstitutionalization. Two extensive reviews of the effects of group treatment underscore the importance of a moderately high degree of social structure. One of these reviews (May, 1976), in which drug treatments are compared to other types of treatment for schizophrenia, concluded that aftercare groups helped patients remain in the community if they focused on such topics as concrete problem-solving, social adjustment, living arrangements, employment and medication compliance, but not when they focused on intensive psychological exploration. A more recent review of 43 studies by Kanas (1986) concluded that "Group therapy was judged to be an effective modality of treatment for schizophrenics in 67% of the inpatient studies [and] . . . 80% of the outpatient studies. Interaction-oriented approaches were more effective than insight-oriented approaches which were found to be harmful for some schizophrenics" (p. 339).

Group Treatment for Borderline Patients

While there has been a good deal of impressionistic clinical evidence in recent years regarding the usefulness of groups for borderline patients (cf. Horwitz, 1980), to date there has been little systematic, empirical research. Preliminary efforts in examining the process and outcome of group treatments for patients with borderline disorders are just now beginning to appear in the literature. A process study by Greene, Rosenkrantz and Muth (1985), for example, found that the borderline patients' views of themselves in the group, in terms of evaluation, potency and activity, were directly related to their perceptions of the group therapists. Kretch, Goren and Wasserman (1987) examined the effects of individual and group psychotherapy for borderline and neurotic patients. Compared to the neurotic patients, borderline patients showed greater improvement over a one year period on several measures of ego functions as a result of their participation in group therapy.

The Structure of Groups

Many of the studies of the effects of group structure have been conducted in the context of day treatment programs. Klyczek and Mann (1986) compared two such programs, one offering twice as much psychotherapy as activity, the other offering twice as much activity therapy. With respect to a wide range of symptoms, the

activity therapy program was found to be significantly more effective. While this same program also yielded a greater rate of relapse
than the program emphasizing psychotherapy, length of stay during
rehospitalization was shorter so that community tenure was equivalent across both programs. In another outcome study, Glick et al.
(1986) compared an intensive day treatment program with a weekly
outpatient therapy group and found no differences on any of their
measures, either at discharge or at 6 and 12 month followups. In an
outcome study of schizophrenic patients, Linn, Caffey, Klett, Hogarty and Lamb (1979) studied ten different day treatment programs
and found that "more professional staff hours, group therapy and a
high patient turnover treatment philosophy were associated with
poor result centers . . . [while] more occupational therapy and a
sustained nonthreatening environment were more characteristic of
successful outcome centers" (p. 1055). One inpatient study by
West et al. (1982) compared an unstructured discussion group with
an activity group and found that both modalities were equivalent in
terms of improving overall adjustment in their sample of heteroge-
neously diagnosed patients.

Three studies were found that explored preferences for specific
kinds of group treatment as a function of psychiatric diagnosis.
Gould and Glick (1976) surveyed patients' preferences for 20 aspects of inpatient treatment. They concluded that "treatment activities emphasizing development of relationships accounted for 38 of
the 40 first ranks, while those activities focusing on other aspects of
the therapeutic milieu such as occupational therapy and community
meetings were ranked last by 34 of the 40 patients. This hierarchy
was essentially independent of diagnosis . . ." (p. 32). A similar
study by Leszcz, Yalom and Norden (1985) obtained essentially
equivalent findings. In this case, group psychotherapy focusing on
here-and-now interactions was the most highly valued modality for
borderline patients, while schizophrenic patients preferred less intensive discussion groups. Both schizophrenic and borderline patients rated occupational therapy low in this study.

The study most closely resembling the present one was conducted by Johnson, Sandel and Bruno (1984). Dance therapy

groups with more or less structure were offered to schizophrenic and character-disordered patients. Results showed that patients with schizophrenia preferred the less structured sessions, while patients with characterological disorders preferred the more highly structured sessions.

Summary

In attempting to summarize these findings, it becomes evident that research on group treatment is an inexact science at best. The variations of groups being offered in a multiplicity of settings with differing treatment philosophies and cultures continue to confound process and outcome studies and make integration of the cumulative findings nearly impossible. Yalom (1983) points out that "we must settle for studies that are less than perfect: either methodologically flawed or performed in different but related clinical settings" (p. 27). Taken as a whole, however, the data do appear to be consistent with his assertion "that inpatient group therapy technique must be modulated to fit the type of patient population: different diagnostic groups require different group therapy approaches" (p. 33). The present study is designed to provide additional empirical validation of this prevailing clinical wisdom.

THE STUDY

Hypotheses

In the context of an inpatient setting offering comparatively unstructured psychotherapy groups and somewhat more structured task-oriented occupational therapy groups to both psychotic and borderline patients, we examined patients' cognitive-affective reactions to their groups, to their leaders, and toward themselves. This preliminary field study was designed to test two specific hypotheses regarding the relationship between levels of psychopathology and group structure. First, an interaction was expected in which borderlines would show more favorable reactions in the unstructured psychotherapy groups, while psychotic patients would respond more favorably in the task-focused occupational therapy groups. A second interaction was expected in which borderline patients would show greater differential reactions to the two kinds of group experiences than psychotic patients.

Method

Setting

This pilot study was performed on an intermediate term psychiatric ward, run as an intensive multimodal treatment unit. At the time of admission, patients are routinely assigned to one of three ongoing psychotherapy groups based on their degree of psychological impairment. Each of these groups is composed of 6 or 7 patients. At the time of this study, a new occupational therapy program was instituted on the ward that included the formation of 12-week task-oriented groups. Three such groups were developed, with patient composition corresponding to the psychotherapy groups. Thus, the same groupings of patients worked together on both psychotherapeutic and occupational therapeutic tasks.

Subjects

Data were collected on a total of 20 patients, all male, ranging in age from 22-69 years. Educational levels varied from 10th grade to 4 years of college. Based on their clinical impressions, the two authors independently classified these patients as either psychotic or borderline. Agreement occurred on all but one case, this being resolved by consensus following a careful review of the clinical record. As a result of these procedures, 11 patients were identified as psychotic and 9 as borderline.

Measures

A six-item semantic differential form, tapping Osgood, Suci and Tannenbaum's (1957) basic factors of evaluation, potency and activity, was used to assess patients' reactions toward the two groups, their leaders and themselves in each group. With the intent of avoiding potentially confounding issues having to do with the formative and terminal phases of group development, this instrument was administered to all patients of the ward during the eighth week of the time-limited occupational therapy groups.

Results

Cell means and standard deviations of patients' ratings are reported in Table 1. To assess the two hypothesized interactions, a series of 2 (psychotic vs. borderline levels of psychopathology) × 2 (psychotherapy vs. task-oriented occupational therapy groups) repeated measures analyses of variance was performed on the semantic differential ratings, using a least squares procedure (Wilkinson, 1986).

Directly pertaining to the first hypothesis are the evaluative ratings of each therapeutic group. It was hypothesized that the borderline patients would more highly value the psychotherapy groups, while the psychotic patients would rate the task-oriented groups more positively. This hypothesized interaction was not empirically substantiated. The data did reveal, however, a significant main ef-

Table 1

Ratings of psychotic- and borderline-level patients in two kinds of groups

Referent	Psychotic				Borderline			
	Psychotherapy		Task-oriented		Psychotherapy		Task-oriented	
	M	SD	M	SD	M	SD	M	SD
Evaluation of group	10.54	3.20	11.45	2.38	8.22	3.52	10.88	2.52
Potency of group	9.54	2.65	10.00	3.13	6.22	4.68	9.88	3.29
Activity of group	9.09	3.70	9.72	2.93	6.77	3.86	10.00	4.03
Evaluation of leader	10.18	4.14	12.09	2.58	5.88	3.68	12.44	2.24
Potency of leader	9.63	1.91	10.00	2.94	6.33	3.20	9.33	2.59
Activity of leader	10.45	2.11	10.20	1.98	7.00	3.90	10.88	2.36
Evaluation of self	9.00	3.57	9.81	2.48	7.66	3.67	7.11	4.78
Potency of self	7.90	3.23	8.72	1.95	9.00	3.96	7.00	4.35
Activity of self	8.54	3.88	10.00	2.32	9.22	3.83	6.55	4.21

fect of kind of group on evaluative ratings. In this clinical setting, the task-oriented occupational therapy groups were more highly regarded than the psychotherapy groups by both psychotic and borderline patients ($p < .05$). Analyses of simple effects revealed that this overall preference was based primarily upon the differential reactions of the borderline patients. Only the borderline patients, not the psychotic patients, showed statistically significant ($p < .05$) differential reactions to the two kinds of groups, a finding that directly supports our second hypothesis.

Perceptions of the potency and activity of the two kinds of groups, as well as attributions of group leadership on all three semantic dimensions, followed this same general pattern. Compared to the psychotherapy groups, the occupational therapy groups tended to be seen as more potent and active and their leaders as significantly more valuable ($p < .05$), potent ($p < .05$), and active ($p < .05$). These findings thus fail to provide support for the first hypothesis. In every instance, however, the analyses of simple effects directly support the second hypothesis of differential sensitivity to the two kinds of group experience. Borderline patients consistently showed statistically significant differential reactions to the groups and their leaders, while the psychotic patients showed no significant differential reactivity across the two group settings.

With respect to self perceptions during group participation, a different pattern of responses emerged. Here, interactive patterns in line with our first hypothesis were obtained. Borderline patients viewed themselves more favorably, in terms of evaluation, potency and activity, when involved in the psychotherapy groups, while the psychotic patients held more favorable self perceptions in the occupational therapy groups. This interaction tended toward statistical significance with regard to perceptions of self activity ($p < .10$).

Discussion

How can these findings be understood? As anticipated, the psychotic patients failed to demonstrate significant differential reactions to the two kinds of group structure on any of the cognitive-affective dimensions tapped. This apparent obliviousness to real differences in the social field may be the result of the operation of the defensive processes of denial and withdrawal and of impairments in attentional processes and capacities for establishing psychological boundaries, phenomena associated with psychotic conditions. To further substantiate this speculation, we conducted ancillary analyses regarding the psychotic patients' relationship to the small group. For each dimension of the semantic differential, we calculated difference scores between ratings of self and the group as a whole and between ratings of self and the group leaders. These scores are considered indices of patients' involvement in or identification with the group; the smaller the difference score, the less the presumed psychological distance between the individual patient and the group or its leader (Greene, Rosenkrantz & Muth, 1985). As expected, *t*-tests on these scores across the two kinds of groups were not significant for the psychotic subsample. That is, the psychotic patients showed no significant differences in their level of involvement across the two small groups. These findings would seem to provide further support for the view of a bland, undifferentiated affective stance by psychotic patients toward the social field.

In contrast to this pattern of response, and supporting our second hypothesis, are the data from the borderline patients. As expected from prevailing theories of borderline psychopathology. these patients reacted in significantly different ways to the two kinds of group. These findings are consistent with the view of the borderline patient as needing to draw heightened and exaggerated boundaries and distinctions. Results of our ancillary analyses of self-group and self-leader difference scores further supported this idea of the borderline patients' keen sensitivity to real differences in the social environment. Unlike the psychotic patients, the borderline patients' connection to the group and its leader clearly depended upon the nature of the group task and structure (self-group difference scores: $t = 2.48, p < .05$, for evaluation; $t = 2.88, p < .05$, for potency; $t = 2.87, p < .05$, for activity; self-leader difference scores: $t = 7.73, p < .001$, for evaluation; $t = 2.29, p = .05$, for potency; $t = 3.85, p < .01$, for activity).

Contrary to our first hypothesis, however, was the directionality of the borderline patients' responses. Unexpectedly, these patients tended to express more favorable reactions for the occupational therapy groups and their leaders. Only with regard to self perceptions did their responses support our initial hypothesis of more posi-

tive reactions during participation in the unstructured psychotherapy groups. The specific pattern of obtained responses by the
borderline patients may have to do with issues of self esteem and
autonomous functioning, considered core themes in borderline psychopathology. As postulated by Masterson (1981), the borderline's
taking initiative and engaging in activity are often associated with a
view of self as bad and unloveable. For the borderline, maintenance
of self esteem requires the renouncing of autonomous activity. Perhaps the requirements of the task-oriented small group, including
decision-making, persuasion and active participation, served to
heighten such pathognomonic conflicts over autonomy. To the extent that autonomous activities are conflictual for borderline patients and are dealt with by splitting processes, it may be that, in
this specific clinical context, they externalized good feelings about
autonomy onto the occupational therapy groups and their leaders
and reserved bad feelings for themselves.

How do these differential reactions of borderline and psychotic
patients affect group process? Leaders who try to develop a specific
structure for groups need to remain aware of differences between
psychotic and borderline patients' defensive and coping styles.
While considerable structuring of groups may be clinically useful
for psychotic patients, these patients may dynamically prefer to dis-
regard distinctions and blur boundaries in the group (cf. Wexler,
Johnson, Geller & Gorden, 1984). In the same vein, while a less
structured atmosphere may be therapeutic for borderline patients,
their preferences for splitting and fragmenting of experience may
dynamically create very rigid artificial divisions and exaggerated
separations within and between groups. In essence, we are positing
an ongoing interplay or tension between the level of structure that
the group leader deems appropriate for accomplishing the task and
the degree of structure defensively needed or desired by the patients.

While the present findings and our speculations need to be read
with considerable caution, given the preliminary nature of this investigation, the limited methodology and the host of potentially
confounding dimensions that occur naturally on an inpatient ward,
occupational therapists should, nevertheless, be encouraged by the
present results. The general preference for the structured activity
groups by both the psychotic and borderline patients would seem to

warrant further investigation of why these groups are valued and how they promote therapeutic change. The specific elements of the activity group, including the use of manual and organizational skills, working on concrete tasks, and choice of project, can be isolated and their effects on psychotic and borderline patients studied in the kind of field study reported here.

A NOTE ON CONFLICTING
FRAMES OF REFERENCE

The theoretical formulations that generated the hypotheses of this study spring from a general psychodynamic framework. That is, the predictions of differential responses of borderline and psychotic patients to varying levels of group structure derived from prevailing psychodynamic understandings of these basic levels of psychopathology. That this is the case should not be surprising, given that the clinical context in which this study was conducted is basically psychodynamically oriented. The inevitable tensions that differing theoretical and therapeutic orientations create on a ward such as this also found their way into the conducting of the present research, the generating of hypotheses and the interpretation of findings. The ongoing challenge, for researchers, as well as clinicians, is to be open to other points of view, including if necessary, yielding or revising one's conceptual framework in the light of new experience. Research such as the present study, conducted by individuals with contrasting frames of reference, while challenging and stressful, at times, provides an important opportunity for creative theoretical integration. Having concrete data at hand, as opposed to clinical dogma, seems to facilitate a collaborative, integrative spirit for furthering our understanding of the therapeutic mechanisms of small groups.

REFERENCES

Burke, J.P. (1983). Defining occupation: Importing and organizing interdisciplinary knowledge. In G. Kielhofner (Ed.), *Health through occupation: Theory and practice in occupational therapy* (pp. 125-138). Philadelphia: F.A. Davis.

Fidler, G. (1969). The task-oriented group as a context for treatment. *American Journal of Occupational Therapy, 23,* 43-48.

Glick, I., Flemming, L., DeChillo, N., Jackson, C., Muscara, D., & Good-Ellis,

M. (1986). A controlled study of transitional day care for non-chronically ill patients. *American Journal of Psychiatry, 143,* 1551-1556.

Gould, E., & Glick, I. (1976). Patient-staff judgements of treatment program helpfulness on a psychiatric ward. *British Journal of Medical Psychology, 49,* 23-33.

Greene, L.R., Rosenkrantz, J., & Muth, D. (1985). Splitting dynamics, self representations and boundary phenomena in the group psychotherapy of borderline personality disorders. *Psychiatry, 48,* 234-245.

Henry, A., Nelson, D., & Duncomb, L. (1984). Choice making in group and individual activity. *American Journal of Occupational Therapy, 38,* 245-251.

Horwitz, L. (1980). Group psychotherapy for borderline and narcissistic patients. *Bulletin of the Menninger Clinic, 44,* 181-200.

Howe, M., & Schwartzberg, S. (1986). *A functional approach to group work in occupational therapy.* Philadelphia: J.B. Lippincott.

Johnson, D., Sandel, S., & Bruno, C. (1984). Effectiveness of different group structures for schizophrenic, character disordered and normal groups. *International Journal of Group Psychotherapy, 34,* 415-429.

Kanas, N. (1986). Group therapy with schizophrenics: A review of controlled studies. *International Journal of Group Psychotherapy, 36,* 339-351.

Kernberg, O. (1976). *Object relations theory and clinical psychoanalysis.* New York: Jason Aronson.

Klyczek, J., & Mann, W. (1986). Therapeutic modality comparisons in day treatment. *American Journal of Occupational Therapy, 40,* 606-611.

Kremer, E., Nelson. D., & Duncomb, L. (1984). Effects of selected activities on affective meaning in psychiatric patients. *American Journal of Occupational Therapy, 38,* 522-528.

Kretch, R., Goren, Y., & Wasserman, A. (1987). Change patterns of borderline patients in individual and group therapy. *International Journal of Group Psychotherapy, 37,* 95-112.

Leszcz, M., Yalom. I., & Norden, M. (1985). The value of inpatient group psychotherapy: Patients' perceptions. *International Journal of Group Psychotherapy, 35,* 411-433.

Linn, M., Caffey, E., Klett, J., Hogarty, G., & Lamb, R. (1979). Day treatment and psychotropic drugs in the aftercare of schizophrenic patients. *Archives of General Psychiatry, 36,* 1055-1066.

Masterson, J. (1981). *The narcissistic and borderline disorders.* New York: Brunner/Mazel.

May, P. (1976). When, what, and why? Psychopharmacotherapy and other treatments in schizophrenia. *Comprehensive Psychiatry, 17,* 683-693.

Osgood, C., Suci, G., & Tannenbaum, P. (1957). *The measurement of meaning.* Urbana, IL: University of Illinois Press.

Rice, C., & Rutan, S. (1987). *Inpatient group psychotherapy: A psychodynamic perspective.* New York: Macmillan.

Schwartzberg, S., Howe, M., & McDermott, A. (1982). A comparison of three treatment group formats for facilitating social interaction. *Occupational Therapy in Mental Health, 2,* 1-16.

Scott, A., & Ross, M. (1987). Present resources as a basis for group dynamics in occupational therapy. In M. Ross (Ed.), *Group process using therapeutic activities in chronic care*. Thorofare, NJ: Slack.

West, E., Jackson, A., Physentides, A., Seenivasagan, S., Jezard, R., Nicholson, A., Ram, R., & Knight, H. (1982). Randomized comparative trial of a ward discussion group. *British Journal of Psychiatry, 141*, 76-80.

Wexler, B., Johnson, D., Geller, J., & Gorden, J. (1984). Group psychotherapy with schizophrenic patients: An example of the oneness group. *International Journal of Group Psychotherapy, 34*, 451-467.

White, R. (1971). The urge towards competence. *American Journal of Occupational Therapy, 25*, 271-274.

Wilkinson, L. (1986). SYSTAT: *The system for statistics*. Evanston, IL: SYSTAT, Inc.

Yalom, I. (1983). *Inpatient group psychotherapy*. New York: Basic Books.

The Effect of Three Group Formats on Group Interaction Patterns

Ardath A. McDermott, MS, OTR/L

SUMMARY. The interaction patterns in task groups, verbal groups, and activity-based verbal groups were compared in order to generate information about the effect of group format on the communication process. The results indicated that the task group formats had more positive social-emotional communications, more interaction between members, and fewer members not interacting than the other two formats. The verbal and activity-based verbal groups had more discussion of feelings and more leader involvement. These findings have usefulness for selecting treatment group formats to best meet therapeutic needs and for validating the distinct role of activity groups within the overall treatment program.

PURPOSE

In selecting group formats to address therapeutic needs of patients, occupational therapists have relied heavily on accumulated

Ardath A. McDermott is the Fieldwork Supervisor and Supervisor of Occupational Therapy in the Adult Admissions Service at Mayview State Hospital, 1601 Mayview Road, Bridgeville, PA 15017. Data collection for this study was done during employment as Assistant Professor at the University of Pittsburgh.

Appreciation is extended to Ramona Monaco, MPH, OTR/L, Director of Westmoreland Partial Hospitalization Program and Chief Occupational Therapist, for making it possible to do this study within her treatment program and for her involvement in implementation of the study. Appreciation is expressed to the staff and clients for their support and cooperation in the project.

Special thanks are extended to Robert R. Conley, MD, Director of Admissions at Mayview State Hospital and Assistant Professor in Psychiatry, University of Pittsburgh School of Medicine, and to Joyce Bell, BS, Research Associate, Western Psychiatric Institute and Clinic, for their central role and support in statistical analysis.

69

experiential knowledge and on formal theory to provide the rationale for structuring interventions. Much of the fundamental conceptualization and interpretation regarding group process was acquired from literature or instruction based on work with insight-oriented verbal groups rather than activity groups. It is reasonable to think that there are fundamental differences between the process of these differing group formats, as well as the therapeutic outcomes.

Need for verification of the theories on which activity groups are based has been discussed both for the importance of developing a scientific basis for group implementation and for conveying its unique therapeutic contribution to other professionals (DeCarlo & Mann, 1985; Mumford, 1974). According to a recent study, 60% of the occupational therapists surveyed used group modalities in their practice, and 76% of the groups described used an activity format or a combination activity and verbal format (Duncombe & Howe, 1985). All of the groups surveyed had more than one goal, the most common being "to increase socialization and communication" (Duncombe & Howe, 1985, p. 169). Thus, use of group treatment modalities is highly prevalent in current occupational therapy practice, which supports the need for clarification of the impact of group format on the communication process. The aim of this study was to further delineate one aspect of the relationship of group structure to outcome by identifying the types of verbal communication and the participants involved in interaction in different group formats.

LITERATURE REVIEW

Much of the literature on group format describes broad benefits of activity-based groups, especially with long-term, chronically ill, psychotic patients. The types of improvements usually include increase in interpersonal involvement, increase in activity level, and improvement in adjustment within the environment. The activity format is thought to be preferable to a verbal format for use with long-term, psychotic patients (Bell, 1970; Leopold, 1976). According to Leopold (1976), the treatment needs of this population are best served by programming graded at varying levels according to the functional levels and needs of the patients.

Other authors shared their observations on the results of instituting therapy groups with activity-based formats. Group projects used to promote interaction and sense of group cohesiveness were found to increase social interaction and involve patients who were usually isolative (Bobis, Harrison, & Traub, 1955; Dunton, 1937; White, 1953). Group projects were also described as bringing about gains in interest and performance level on tasks (White, 1953) and improvement in functional level and readiness for community living (Bobis et al., 1955).

Group programs including a range of social activities were found to be successful in helping patients to socialize in normal ways, to become more involved with others, to improve behavioral consistency, and to learn adaptive coping skills (Bell, 1970; Hyde, York, & Wood, 1948; Koven & Shuff, 1953; Lockerbie & Stevenson, 1947; Mallinson & Lawson, 1957; Pasewark & Hornby, 1968; Webb, 1973). A program of daily groups including verbal therapy, recreation, socialization, reading, music, or crafts enabled chronic patients characterized as apathetic to become more active, more sociable, and more expressive of their opinions in group sessions (Springfield & Tullis, 1958). In a carefully designed group program including a planning phase, an activity phase, and an evaluation phase, patients were able to achieve maximal group involvement and learn about finding satisfaction in group participation (Howe, 1968). Activity-based verbal formats and parallel task formats focusing on identification of emotions were found to be effective in helping patients acquire an awareness of emotions necessary for communication with others (Angel, 1981). Throughout this report, the phrase, activity-based verbal groups, will be used to refer to formats combining awareness-oriented activities and discussion.

Others have compared the effect of using different types of group formats on the interaction patterns in treatment groups. The first set of comparison studies dealt with low-functioning patients, including those with schizophrenic or other chronically debilitating psychiatric illnesses. In parallel task groups, addition of a break for smoking and conversing resulted in significantly higher ratings on an instrument measuring social interaction, general behavior, and task performance than in the control group which had no such break (Olson & Sherman, 1961). In three studies comparing parallel task and project group formats with chronic schizophrenic patients, two

of the studies showed significantly greater increases in social interaction with the project group format (Levine, Marks, & Hall, 1957;
Werner, Maddigan, & Watson, 1969), while the other study showed
no difference (Efron, Marks, & Hall, 1959). Comparing a project
group and an activity-based verbal group with schizophrenic patients, there was no significant difference in amount of interaction
during the activities, but there was a trend toward more verbalization in the discussion period after the project group than in the period after the activity-based verbal group (Odhner, 1970). Amount
of interaction was compared in group programs with graded levels
of structure for a chronic schizophrenic population (Beal, Duckro,
Elias, & Hecht, 1977). Greater increases in interaction were found
with increasing degrees of structure in the group treatment programs. Thus, with the chronic schizophrenic population, project
group formats and maximal structure appear to provide the optimal
conditions for facilitating socialization.

Studies have also looked at the effect of group format on interaction patterns with relatively higher-functioning, non-psychotic individuals. In an acute-care setting with primarily non-psychotic patients, the amount and type of verbal interaction were compared in a
parallel task format, an activity-based verbal group, and a verbal
group (Schwartzberg, Howe, & McDermott, 1982). Sociograms
and a modification of the Bales System of Interaction Process Analysis (Bales, 1950a) were used to tabulate the number of interactions
of each type in representative segments of the group. Among the
significant findings, the parallel task group had more interactions
between members, more total interaction, and fewer non-communicating members. There were also more questions about suggestions, information, and feelings, and a trend toward more positive
social-emotional comments than in the other two formats. The activity-based verbal group and the verbal group formats had significantly more comments, by both members and leaders, to the whole
group and more non-communicating members than the task groups.
The verbal group had more non-communicating members than both
of the activity-based formats. It was suggested that this information
be used in differentially prescribing group treatment formats which
would best address the individual's social skill deficits and needs.

The same comparisons were made in five activity group formats with occupational therapy students in a group process course (McDermott & Wolfe, 1984). No significant differences were found in interaction patterns. It appeared that variations in group format had no differential effect with the student groups, because the students did not have the social skill deficits characteristic of most psychiatric patients.

Other relationships between group format and outcome have been studied. Comparing cooperative and competitive formats for facilitating interaction among emotionally-disturbed children, the cooperative format was found to be the most effective (Fahl, 1970). Activity-based, awareness-oriented verbal groups were found to be more effective than purely verbal groups for developing interpersonal skills (DeCarlo & Mann, 1985; Mumford, 1974). Including structured group activities in day treatment programs was shown to have positive effects on treatment outcomes (Klyczek & Mann, 1986; Linn, Caffey, Klett, Hogarty, & Lamb, 1979).

Several inferences can be drawn from these observations and research findings. With a schizophrenic population, socialization and development of social skills appears to be enhanced by use of group projects, by inclusion of a discussion segment in task groups, and by socialization activities graded according to the patients' levels. With higher functioning, non-psychotic patients, task groups promote peer interaction with a strong element of emotionally positive tone. Activity-based verbal groups are useful for improving social skills, learning to speak to a group, and minimizing the chance of social withdrawal within the group. Unstructured verbal groups facilitate speaking to a group as a whole. Thus, the unique value of activity in treatment groups is clearly illustrated in these findings.

METHOD

A descriptive research method was used to study and compare the patterns of verbal interaction in eight treatment group formats. These formats were later combined into three categories for purposes of data analysis, with two group formats being eliminated. The formats are listed here by category:

Verbal Groups:
  Theme Group
  Contemporary Issues Group
Activity-Based Verbal Groups:
  Mental Health Seminar
  Self-Awareness Group
Task Groups:
  Ceramics Group
  Art Group

The verbal category included formats consisting of discussion only. The activity-based verbal groups focused discussion on an activity, such as structured awareness exercises, values clarification exercises, or reading pertinent articles together. Task groups followed primarily a parallel task format with members working on individual projects in the same area.

The treatment setting was a partial hospital program in a community mental health center. The subjects attended the program two days each week and were likely to be in a combination of several of the eight groups studied. Four of the eight groups occurred on each of the days these patients attended, and all eight groups were observed each week. A series of five observation sequences was conducted over a period of five weeks, with all groups occurring in each observation sequence. Group observations were conducted by recording the interaction patterns in segments of each group on a sociogram. Within each group, two 5-minute segments were observed, beginning at 15 minutes and 25 minutes past the beginning of the hour-long groups. These segments were assumed to be representative of interaction patterns throughout the entire session. Each interaction was categorized according to a modified form of the Bales Interaction Process Analysis Method, indicating the type of interaction (Bales, 1950a, 1950b). The use of sociograms (Bradford, Stock, & Horwitz, 1978; Hearn, 1978; Howe & Schwartzberg, 1986) and the Bales System of categorizing interactions (Benjamin, 1978; Golembiewski, 1962; Howe & Schwartzberg, 1986; Sampson & Marthas, 1977) have been described as useful ways of observing and analyzing a group's communication structure. The recordings were tabulated to show amount of interaction, type of interaction, and participants in interaction for each segment observed.

A modified form of the Bales System has been used successfully by this investigator in the previously cited study by Schwartzberg, Howe, and McDermott (1982). For this study, it was amended to include communications which were noted to occur during its prior use, but were not indicated in the Bales System. The amended version is shown in Table 1. Additions of interaction types 5/6 and 7/8 were made to represent comments including both factual information and feelings in one statement and questions which addressed both information and feelings. The category, "asking for equipment," was necessary to categorize such comments occurring regularly in task groups. A category was added for group laughter, because this seemed to represent an important indicator of the nature of the communication. Each unit of interaction noted refers to one individual's comment from beginning to end with no intervening statement by another group participant.

Data was collected by a participant observer seated on the periphery of the group. The observer attended the groups for two weeks prior to beginning data collection in order to decrease the effect of the observer's presence on group interaction patterns during the study. The nature and purpose of the study was explained to all patients in the program with emphasis on the fact that the focus of the study was the group process, not the nature or content of any individual's participation. Explanation was provided and a consent form was signed prior to their attendance at any group where observations were taking place.

Variables which could have affected the interaction patterns were tabulated on a log for each group session. The information recorded included a code number for each patient present, the number of patients in the session, the number of patients with each diagnosis, ages, COTE scores, the activity chosen, and special events happening concurrently within the treatment setting. Each patient was assigned a code number, which was used in recording of the sociogram and group log. Thus, descriptive data needed for the log and subsequent demographic data analysis could be kept by patient code

Table 1

Categories of Interaction Adapted from the Bales System

A. Positive social-emotional comments: 1. Gives compliment

                                          2. Jokes, shows satisfaction

                                          3. Agrees, shows understanding

B. Task-oriented statements: 4. Gives suggestion or direction

                                          5. Expresses feeling or opinion

                                          6. Gives information

                                        5/6. States information and feelings

C. Task-oriented questions: 7. Asks for information

                                          8. Asks about feelings or opinions

                                          9. Asks for suggestion or direction

                                        7/8. Asks for information and feelings

D. Negative social-emotional comments: 10. Disagrees, shows rejection

                                         11. Shows frustration, asks for help

                                         12. Shows antagonism, criticizes

Eq. Asks for equipment

L. Group laughter

Participants in interactions: M-M. Member to member

                                        M-G. Member to group

                                        M-L. Member to leader

                                        L-M. Leader to member

                                        L-G. Leader to group

                                        L-L. Leader to leader

                                         NT. Member not talking

                                        NTT. Member not talked to

                                         NC. Member not talking or talked to

---

numbers, in order to obscure identifying data about individuals. The diagnostic categories were Affective Disorders, Anxiety Disorders, Schizophrenic Disorders, and Other Disorders. The latter category included Personality Disorders, Adjustment Disorders, and Substance Use Disorders. The COTE score is a rating on the Comprehensive Occupational Therapy Evaluation, which indicates level of functioning in general behavior, task performance, and social skills (Brayman, Kirby, Misenheimer, & Short, 1976). Individual COTE scores calculated for each day of attendance were averaged for each group to determine a general functional level for the group.

RESULTS

The interaction patterns in the eight groups observed were compared using two-way analysis of variance by the Mann-Whitney U formula. The statistical analysis of the eight formats showed inconsistent findings with broad variability between demographic characteristics and communication patterns. In order to bring the data analysis into clearer focus, the groups were categorized into three types of formats according to similarities in group structure. Two groups were eliminated to allow for equal numbers of group formats in each category. The two groups eliminated were chosen because one had extremely small patient numbers, and the other did not adequately conform to any of the designated categories. The analysis of variance was used to identify significant differences among the three group formats in demographic characteristics, number of occurrences of each type of interaction, and members involved in interaction. When a significant difference among the groups was shown to be present, identification of the pairs of groups in which the means of groups differed significantly was achieved using the Neuman-Keuls procedure, an a posteriori test for multiple comparisons.

Comparison of group demographic data showed some differences between the three formats, as shown in Table 2. The number of patients ranged from 2 to 16, and the mean was significantly higher in the activity-based verbal groups than in the task groups. With an age range of 23 to 42 years old, the mean age was significantly higher in the activity-based verbal groups than in the task groups.

Table 2

Variations in Group Characteristics

| Characteristic | Group Formats | | | | | | ANOVA | Newman-Keuls Comparison | | |
| | Verbal(V) | | Activity/Verbal(A/V) | | TASK(T) | | | Groups compared | | |
	M	SD	M	SD	M	SD	F	V&A/V	V&T	A/V&T
Number of patients	7.90	4.72	12.70	2.67	5.60	1.78	12.08	*	-	***
Age	36.20	4.98	36.70	2.21	31.20	5.88	4.31	-	-	*
COTE score	87.20	4.26	83.20	4.42	85.70	5.72	1.74	-	-	-
Schizophrenic Disorders	0.10	0.32	0.30	0.48	0.50	0.53	1.96	-	-	-
Affective Disorders	4.90	4.12	8.60	2.07	2.10	0.88	14.48	*	*	***
Anxiety Disorders	2.30	0.95	1.90	0.99	1.70	1.06	0.93	-	-	-
Other Disorders	0.60	0.52	1.90	0.88	1.30	0.48	10.03	***	**	-

Note. * = $p < .05$ - = Not significant

** = $p < .01$ M = Mean

*** = $p < .001$ SD = Standard deviation

There were significant differences in the number of patients with Affective Disorders among all the groups, with the most occurring in the activity-based verbal groups and the fewest in the task groups. The verbal groups had significantly fewer patients with a diagnosis classified as Other Disorders than the activity-based verbal and task groups.

Comparing the number of occurrences of each type of interaction showed the task groups to have significantly more communications than the other two formats in the categories of giving compliments (1), joking or showing satisfaction (2), positive social-emotional comments (A), and member-to-member interaction (MM). Task groups also had more offering of suggestions or direction (4), showing frustration or asking for help (11), and asking for equipment (Eq). These findings are shown in Tables 3 and 4. The activity-based verbal groups and the verbal groups had significantly more interactions than the task groups in the categories of asking about and expressing opinions or feelings (5,8), leader-to-group comments (LG), members not talking (NT), members not talked to (NTT), and members not actively involved in communication, either by talking or being talked to (NC). The task format had significantly more requests for information (7) than the activity-based verbal format. The activity-based verbal format had less stating of information (6) than the task and verbal formats. The total amount of interaction did not differ significantly between the three formats. This eliminated the concern that the actual amount of each type of interaction would represent a different portion of the total group process if the total amount of interaction differed between formats. Comparisons of the findings with the most value for practical application are illustrated in Figure 1.

In order to rule out variance in the demographic variables as contributing factors in the findings of differences between the formats, the group interaction patterns were analyzed by each of the demographic variables which varied significantly between formats. Those demographic variables were patient number, number of Affective Disorders, number of Other Disorders, and mean age. Two-way analysis of variance showed significant variance in some communication types with patient number, number of Affective Disorders, and mean age, but not with number of Other Disorders.

Table 3

Comparison of Types of Interactions Showing Significant Variations Between Group Formats

Type of Interaction	Group Formats Verbal(V)		Group Formats Activity/Verbal(A/V)		TASK(T)		ANOVA	Newman-Keuls Comparison Groups compared		
	M	SD	M	SD	M	SD	F	V&A/V	V&T	A/V&T
1. Gives compliment	0.40	0.97	1.50	2.51	4.70	3.09	8.92	–	***	*
2. Jokes, shows satisfaction	4.50	6.50	3.00	2.94	21.50	11.00	18.43	–	***	***
4. Gives direction	1.30	2.50	2.70	3.13	9.70	8.14	7.39	–	**	*
5. Expresses feeling/opinion	24.40	10.01	24.50	10.22	11.80	6.29	6.55	–	**	**
6. Gives information	33.20	28.65	12.50	11.17	42.20	24.19	4.54	*	–	**
7. Asks for information	12.20	11.33	7.40	7.28	18.90	8.29	4.00	–	–	**
8. Asks for feeling/opinion	6.90	5.95	10.00	8.54	1.80	2.04	4.57	–	*	**
11. Shows frustration	0.00	0.00	0.00	0.00	0.50	0.71	5.00	–	*	*
Eq. Asks for equipment	0.00	0.00	0.00	0.00	1.20	1.55	6.00	–	*	*
A. Positive social-emotional	18.30	14.64	17.00	10.75	35.20	16.50	5.14	–	*	**

Note.   * = p < .05   – = Not significant

   ** = p < .01   M = Mean

   *** = p < .001   SD = Standard deviation

Table 4

Comparison of Participants In Interactions Showing Significant Variations Between Group Formats

| Type of Interaction | Group Formats | | | | | | ANOVA | Newman-Keuls Comparison | | |
| | Verbal(V) | | Activity/ Verbal(A/V) | | TASK(T) | | | Groups compared | | |
	M	SD	M	SD	M	SD	F	V&A/V	V&T	A/V&T
MM. Member to member	12.80	10.81	9.40	8.29	53.30	36.61	11.73	-	**	**
LG. Leader to Group	18.90	18.05	7.80	3.82	2.20	2.74	6.23	-	**	**
NT. Not talking	4.80	4.71	8.00	5.58	0.70	0.82	7.44	-	*	***
NTT. Not talked to	6.20	6.03	8.80	6.44	0.90	1.10	6.15	-	*	**
NC. Not communicating	4.80	4.71	7.90	5.45	0.70	0.82	7.45	-	*	***

Note.   * = $p < .05$ - = Not significant

     ** = $p < .01$ M = Mean

     *** = $p < .001$ SD = Standard deviation

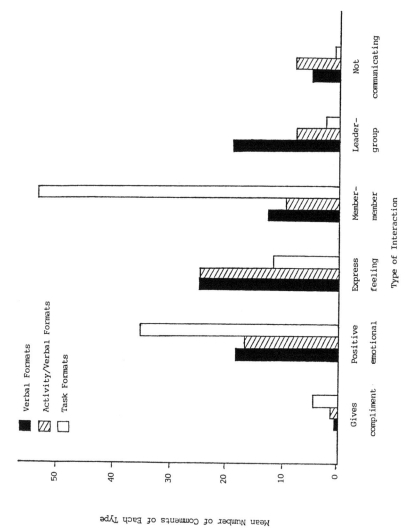

FIGURE 1. Comparison of primary communication differences between group formats

Paired linear regressions were done, based on the Pearson product moment coefficient of correlation (Pearson *r*), to determine which of the significant findings in the ANOVA represented true relationships between the demographic variables and the interaction patterns. Results showed that the members not talking, members not talked to, and non-communicating members increased with the number of patients, the number of Affective Disorders and the relative portion of the group with Affective Disorders. There was also a strongly positive correlation between the number of patients and the number of Affective Disorders ($r = .96, p < .001$), and between the number of patients and the relative portion of the group with Affective Disorders ($r = .72, p < .001$). Mean age was somewhat correlated with number of Affective Disorders ($r = .34, p = .06$). A trend toward more member-to-member interaction occurred in the medium-size groups (6 to 8 members), as compared with the smaller groups (2 to 5 members) or larger groups (11 to 16 members).

DISCUSSION

The results of this study indicate that variations in group format do have an effect on interaction patterns. Beneficial aspects of the task group format were identified. The high occurrence of peer interaction and the low number of members not actively communicating in the task groups reflect the value of task groups for decreasing social isolation and promoting practice of social skills among patients. Task groups were also characterized by more complimenting, joking, and showing satisfaction. Perhaps the task situation promotes exchange of positive comments, creating a comfortable environment which enables patients to interact spontaneously. The presence of a task can provide a non-threatening focus for comments for individuals with difficulty interacting. The prevalence of complimentary statements have relevance for the long-standing conviction that task groups are useful for building self-esteem.

It is logical to find more instances of requesting information, of giving directions, and of asking for equipment in a task group. There, patients are often doing unfamiliar activities for which they need procedural information and direction. Creating the necessity for such interactions is one of the ways occupational therapists have structured therapeutic sessions to promote interaction.

The occurrence of more expression of tension and asking for help in the task group raises some question about the categorization of this type of communication in a negative social-emotional context. Usually, being able to ask for assistance and ventilate frustration in a constructive manner are considered to be adaptive skills for living, which patients are encouraged to learn. Bales' system combines three behaviors in this category: "Shows tension, asks for help, withdraws out of field" (Bales, 1950b, p. 258). This categorization is probably not suitable for this type of study since it does not concur conceptually with the therapeutic principles mentioned. Another consideration in the interpretation of this finding is that this type of interaction occurred only six times in the 30 groups observed, each instance being in a task group. Perhaps, its occurrence only in task groups has statistical significance, but not practical significance. Considering these factors, task groups may actually be useful in helping patients learn to actively and directly seek assistance in getting their needs met.

Distinct patterns were found in the communication processes of the verbal groups and activity-based verbal groups. They had more communication dealing with feelings and information, reflecting the value of verbal groups for learning to verbally express and deal with feelings. A greater portion of the interactions involved the leader speaking to the whole group, indicating the leader role is more central to the on-going group process of the verbal group and the activity-based verbal group. These formats also had more members not actively involved in communication. This may be related to the situation whereby the verbal group format allows for only one person talking at a time, while multiple conversations can be going on simultaneously in a task group.

Confounding factors introduced by the effects of the demographic variables may have contributed to the findings of more non-communicating members in the verbal and activity-based verbal formats. The activity-based verbal groups had significantly more members than the other formats, and the number of non-communicating members was found to increase with the number of patients in the group. With large groups, lack of involvement in communication can result from intimidation about speaking to a large number of people or merely from less chance for all present to speak within a given time period. Optimal group size is often recommended to be from six to eight patients, and this group size showed a trend toward having the most member interaction.

The relative portion of the group members with Affective Disorders appeared to be a factor, also. The activity-based verbal groups had significantly more Affective Disorders than the verbal groups, and both had more than the task groups. The number of non-communicating patients was found to increase with an increase in prevalence of Affective Disorders in the group. The phenomenon of decreased interaction is often experienced by therapists in terms of the effort needed to facilitate interaction in groups with a high number of depressed individuals. No doubt, group size and predominance of Affective Disorders contributed to the finding of more non-communicating participants in the verbal and activity-based verbal formats.

The activity-based verbal groups had significantly fewer occurrences of statements of information than the other formats. In looking over the data, the activity-based verbal groups had less total communication than the other formats. It showed slightly more communication in several categories than the verbal format resulting in a more evenly distributed representation of more types of communication. Though none of these differences reached statistical significance, they may have combined to result in significantly less communications of this one type than in the other formats.

An important consideration in this study is that there was no mechanism for a control group. Since subjects in each group were in a number of the other groups, interaction patterns were, to some extent, an outcome of the combination of groups they were in, with some unique manifestations occurring as a differential effect of each format studied.

Comparing the findings of this study with the results of a similar study done by Schwartzberg, Howe, and McDermott (1983), this study supports some of the earlier findings. In both studies, the task groups had more member interaction and fewer non-communicating members than the other two formats. In this study, the verbal and activity-based verbal groups had more discussion of feelings and opinions than the task format. Similarly, in the previous study, the verbal and activity-based verbal formats had more discussion of feelings, information and suggestions. They concur on the more active role of the leader and the relatively higher occurrence of non-communicating members in the verbal and activity-based verbal formats. This study showed significantly more positive social-emotional comments in the task group, substantiating the pattern which appeared as a trend in the previous study.

Other findings of the two studies did not match. Some of the more interesting findings of the earlier study which were not replicated in this study were more leader-to-member comments and a higher total amount of communication in the task groups. The activity-based verbal format and verbal format had more member comments to the group, more strongly suggesting their value for helping patients learn to speak to a whole group. Also, the activity-based verbal format had fewer non-communicating members than the verbal format, indicating greater effectiveness of the activity-based groups in assuring member involvement. In this study, there were fewer contrasts in the communication patterns between the verbal and the activity-based verbal formats than in the previous study. Discussion of the disparity in findings for the same group formats in different settings raises the important consideration that the interaction patterns in a given format are likely to be greatly affected by the individual leader's approach to structuring and facilitating interaction.

CONCLUSIONS

These results point to some distinctions in the treatment uses of activity and verbal group formats. The task groups are effective in maximizing socialization in a mutually positive exchange, with humor, affirmation, and task-related interactions being a predominant part of the group process. The verbal and activity-based verbal groups are useful for dealing with feelings, opinions, and related information. Attention is also drawn to the need for effort on the part of leader to involve all group members in interaction in groups which do not by nature of their structure assure each member's participation. These findings offer information clarifying one aspect of the contributions of different group formats in providing comprehensive treatment.

These research results are potentially useful in a number of ways. They can provide guidelines for program planning and for planning group sessions specifically geared to the program objectives and patient population. They can be used in assigning individual patients to groups by considering which group format is likely to best achieve that patient's goals. Furthermore, the information can be used to substantiate the therapeutic value of activity groups provided by occupational therapy as a means of supporting the need to expand programming and staffing patterns.

This study examined only one aspect of treatment group outcomes. Further research is needed to clarify other aspects of treatment outcome relative to group format, and a few areas with potential research value are suggested by this study. Activity-based verbal groups have been shown to be useful in building social skills with non-psychotic individuals; and task groups, in facilitating their socialization. Thus, a program incorporating both formats might prove effective by giving them opportunities to learn more about interpersonal skills in structured awareness exercises and practice those skills in task groups. Therapeutic outcomes of this and other group combinations warrant investigation. It would also be useful to explore the amount and type of interaction in different group formats with a schizophrenic population, as this study did with a non-psychotic population. According to reports in the literature, chronic schizophrenic individuals differ from non-psychotic individuals in their responses to various group treatment approaches. Thus, similar investigations in diverse treatment settings would be useful to further clarify the value of different group formats for optimally addressing specific deficits, needs and objectives.

REFERENCES

Angel, S. L. (1981). The emotion identification group. *American Journal of Occupational Therapy, 35*(4), 256-262.

Bales, R. F. (1950a). *Interaction process analysis: A method for the study of small groups.* Cambridge: Addison-Wesley Press.

Bales, R. F. (1950b). A set of categories for the analysis of small group interaction. *American Sociological Review, 15,* 257-468.

Beal, D., Duckro, P., Elias, J., & Hecht, E. (1977). Graded group procedures for long term regressed schizophrenics. *Journal of Nervous and Mental Disease*, *164*(2), 102-106.

Bell, R. W. (1970). Activity as a tool in group therapy. *Perspectives in Psychiatric Care*, *8*(2), 84-91.

Benjamin, A. (1978). *Behavior in Small Groups*. Boston, MA: Houghton Mifflin.

Bobis, B. R., Harrison, R. M., & Traub, L. (1955). Activity group therapy. *American Journal of Occupational Therapy*, *9*(1), 19-21, 50.

Bradford, L. P., Stock, D., & Horwitz, M. (1978). How to diagnose group problems. In Leland, P. B. (Ed.), *Group Development* (2nd ed.). (pp. 62-78). San Diego, CA: University Associates.

Brayman, S. J., Kirby, T. F., Misenheimer, A. M., & Short, M. J. (1976). Comprehensive occupational therapy evaluation scale. *American Journal of Occupational Therapy*, *30*(2), 94-100.

DeCarlo, J. J. & Mann, W. C. (1985). The effectiveness of verbal versus activity groups in improving self-perceptions of interpersonal communication skills. *American Journal of Occupational Therapy*, *39*(1), 20-27.

Duncombe, L. W. & Howe, M. C. (1985). Group work in occupational therapy: a survey of practice. *American Journal of Occupational Therapy*, *39*(3), 163-170.

Dunton, W. R. (1937). Quilt making as a socializing measure. *Occupational Therapy and Rehabilitation*, *16*(4), 275-278.

Efron, H. Y., Marks, H. K., & Hall, R. (1959). A comparison of group centered and individual-centered activity programs. *Archives of General Psychiatry*, *1*(5), 120/552-123/555.

Fahl, M. A. (1970). Emotionally disturbed children: effects of cooperative and competitive activity on peer interaction. *American Journal of Occupational Therapy*, *24*(1), 31-33.

Golembiewski, R. T. (1962). *The Small Group: An Analysis of Research Concepts and Operations*. Chicago, IL: University of Chicago Press.

Hearn, G. (1978). Small group behavior and development: a selective bibliography. In Leland, P. B. (Ed.), Group Development (2nd ed.). (pp. 211-234). San Diego, CA: University Associates Press.

Howe, M. C. (1968). An occupational therapy activity group. *American Journal of Occupational Therapy*, *22*(3), 176-179.

Howe, M. C. & Schwartzberg, S. L. (1986). *A Functional Approach to Group Work in Occupational Therapy*. Philadelphia, PA: Lippincott.

Hyde, R. W., York, R., & Wood, A. C. (1948). Effectiveness of games in a mental hospital. *Occupational Therapy and Rehabilitation*, *27*(4), 304-308.

Klyczek, J. P. & Mann, W. C. (1986). Therapeutic modality comparisons in day treatment. *American Journal of Occupational Therapy*, *40*(9), 606-611.

Koven, B. & Shuff, F. L. (1953). Group therapy with the chronically ill. *American Journal of Occupational Therapy*, *7*(5), 208-219.

Leopold, H. S. (1976). Selective group approaches with psychotic patients in hospital settings. *American Journal of Psychotherapy*, *30*, 95-102.

Levine, D., Marks, H.K., & Hall, R. (1957). Differential effect of factors in an activity therapy program. *American Journal of Psychiatry*, Dec. 532-535.

Linn, M. W., Caffey, E. M., Klett, C. J., Hogarty, G. E., & Lamb, H. R. (1979). Day treatment and psychotropic drugs in the aftercare of schizophrenic patients. *Archives of General Psychiatry*, *36*, 1055-1066.

Lockerbie, L. & Stevenson, G. H. (1947). Socialization through occupational therapy. *Occupational Therapy and Rehabilitation*, *26*(3), 142-145.

Mallinson, T. J. & Lawson, W. T. (1957). Assessing the use of group methods in rehabilitating the psychiatric patient. *Canadian Psychiatric Association Journal*, *2*(4), 190-197.

McDermott, A. A. & Wolfe, C. M. (1984). [Effect of Group Format on Interaction Patterns in Student Groups]. Unpublished raw data.

Mumford, M. S. (1974). A comparison of interpersonal skills in verbal and activity groups. *American Journal of Occupational Therapy*, *28*(5), 281-283.

Odhner, F. (1970). A study of group tasks as facilitators of verbalization among hospitalized schizophrenic patients. *American Journal of Occupational Therapy*, *24*(1), 7-12.

Olson, A. R. & Sherman, L. J. (1961). The effect of planned socialization on patients. *American Journal of Occupational Therapy*, *15*(3), 118-120.

Pasewark, R. & Hornby, R. (1968). The effect upon social interaction patterns of a short-term stimulation program for psychiatric geriatric patients. *American Journal of Occupational Therapy*, *22*(3), 195-196.

Sampson, E. E. & Marthas, M. (1977). *Group Process for the Health Professions* (2nd ed.). New York: Wiley & Sons.

Schwartzberg, S. L., Howe, M. C., & McDermott, A. A. (1982). A comparison of three treatment group formats for facilitating social interaction. *Occupational Therapy in Mental Health*, *2*(4), 1-16.

Springfield, F. B. & Tullis, L. H. (1958). An intensive activities program for chronic neuropsychiatric patients. *American Journal of Occupational Therapy*, *12*(5), 247-249.

Webb, L. J. (1973). The therapeutic social club. *American Journal of Occupational Therapy*, *27*(2), 81-83.

Werner, V., Maddigan, R. F., & Watson, C. G. (1969). A study of two treatment group programs for chronic mentally ill patients in occupational therapy. *American Journal of Occupational Therapy*, *23*(2), 132-136.

White, C. V. (1953). Group projects with psychiatric patients. *American Journal of Occupational Therapy*, *7*(6), 253, 270.

The Process of Group Treatment with the Chronically Mentally Ill

Karla W. Weaver, OTR/L

SUMMARY. Group treatment has been used with inpatient psychiatric clients for numerous years. Only since the advent of deinstitutionalization have outpatient services begun to utilize this format. Over the years, mental health professionals have realized that traditional talk therapy approaches do not adequately address the multiple, pressing needs presented by the person with chronic mental illness. A multi-modality approach that utilizes case management, medication, family support, and group therapy has evolved. Specifically, activity focused group therapy has been recognized as an integral treatment modality. The author presents a model of group treatment and process which underscores the value of Occupational Therapy's contribution to the treatment of the chronically mentally ill.

INTRODUCTION

Agency administrators have long been urging therapists to utilize group treatment because it is cost-effective. Therapists with large caseloads have formed groups of clients demonstrating similar symptoms to enable them to see as many people as frequently as possible. Only in recent years have community mental health services seriously assessed the use of group treatment with the chronically mentally ill. This shift has been due, in part, to the increased emphasis on community treatment as an alternative to hospitalization.

The chronically mentally ill client poses a dilemma for commu-

---

Karla W. Weaver, resides in Yakima, WA, and is affiliated with the Mountain Vista Nursing Home, Toppenish, WA.

nity mental health centers. Often, the client is unable to attend group on a consistent basis and requires much intervention outside the group time. The attention deficits and psychotic symptoms related to thought disorders are disruptive and, frequently, unresponsive in traditional, insight-oriented, highly verbal groups. Limited availability of funding to support the frequent interventions demanded by the chronically mentally ill furthers the agency's dilemma.

Activity groups that met once a week were once thought to be the solution to these problems. Groups of this nature focused on the social deficits of the chronically mentally ill. Clients were encouraged to come together for an hour of leisure activity and establish social relationships. Gradually, activities of these groups changed to include daily living tasks such as cooking and shopping.

Leaders of these groups found that, contrary to the hypothesis, group members did not form social bonds that were continued outside the group. There was little carry-over of information from one group session to the next. Sessions of one hour were determined to be too brief to adequately complete most daily living skill activities.

From these experiences evolved the concept of day treatment. Group members participated in activities lasting up to eight hours, as often as five days a week. Initially, day treatment programs followed the educational model. Group members were assigned to small groups and staff "instructed" them on a variety of topics. Most of the instruction was conducted in the small groups though the entire program met together at least daily to encourage a sense of community. Staff found that group members were more responsive and less overtly psychotic when they were involved in the "classes" that required active physical participation on the part of the members. Gradually more task oriented activities became the norm in day treatment programs. Daily living skills and vocational aspects are not included in most programs of this nature. The sense of community was formalized by Fountain House through the Clubhouse model of day treatment. This model continues to utilize small groups within the framework of the larger group or club. The smaller groups each have a primary function which is needed for the club to continue to operate. In this way, each member of the club contributes to the operation and continuance of the club (Fountain House, 1985).

Numerous variations of the Clubhouse model have arisen as community mental health staff have adapted the structure and techniques to day treatment programs and funding sources in their own communities across the country. The perspective of group treatment of the chronically mentally ill client presented in this article is one such variation.

In this article, one session of group treatment is described and explained. The model presented is applicable to both distinct, infrequent groups and to the sequential programming of day treatment. Emphasis is placed on the process of treatment and the role of the Occupational Therapist in this process. Group goals, structure, and tasks are addressed as they are integral components of the treatment process.

GROUP GOALS

Thought disorders interrupt the ability of the individual to accurately receive and process information from the environment. The resulting distorted view produces distorted behavior (Crabtree, 1984). Treatment seeks to reduce the distortions and enable the chronically mentally ill person to interact on a socially acceptable level within the community (Ely, 1985). Areas which must be addressed if this goal is to be realized include object relations, reality testing, problem solving, socialized behavior, community awareness, self care, and many others (Pepper & Rylewicz, 1984; Crabtree, 1984).

GROUP STRUCTURE

Structure is the cornerstone of group work with the chronically mentally ill. The client's reality is often so fragmented and distorted that external structure is welcomed (Yalom, 1983). A structured group allows the client to function within well defined parameters and provides a sense of predictability in an otherwise unpredictable world.

The most basic form of structure the therapist can provide is a routine within which the group operates. When the same format is used at each session, the client is better able to interpret the group as being reliable and make internal predictions about what will occur. This reliability increases the client's sense of control over both the external and internal environments (Yalom, 1983).

When considering which format to use with any group, the therapist must consider the areas that the formats under consideration address. Whether or not the areas addressed are in keeping with the needs of the group members and how learned skills will be generalized to situations outside the group also need to be evaluated (Yalom, 1983; Ely, 1985).

Five basic phases in the process of effective activity focused group work have been identified by the author. The group tasks and processes are distinctly different as the group progresses through the gathering, grouping, task, process, and planning segments. These differences require that the therapist assume a variety of roles (Pepper & Rylewicz, 1984) to enable the process to be effectively completed.

GROUP TASKS AND PROCESS

The tasks of each group segment help to determine the roles that the therapist assumes during that time. Concurrently, the roles of the therapist affect the process of the segment. It is the therapist's responsibility to assist the group members to improve their individual abilities to function within the group and the community (Ely, 1985). To that end, the primary role adopted by the therapist is that of Enabler. This role takes on many forms as the group moves from one segment of the group format to another.

Gathering

This process begins wherever two group members meet, be it in the parking lot or agency reception area, and continues into the group. It typically includes such activities as exchanging greetings, exploring the room, brief summaries of "what's new," and establishing a position or location within the room. If rest rooms or refreshments are available, these are incorporated into the ritual.

The gathering ritual is vital for group members (Pepper & Rylewicz, 1984). It allows them to become oriented to each other and the environment in which they associate. It distinguishes the therapeutic relationship from others and, by association, the behaviors within the group from those outside (Ely, 1985). This process lays the groundwork for the behavioral and interactional changes that are the goals of treatment (Yalom, 1983).

The therapist must anticipate and accept this phase as an integral part of the group process. The first few minutes of the session may be designated for gathering, or the group meeting area may be available to members prior to the starting time. If the latter option is chosen, the therapist should join the group at least five minutes prior to the beginning of the group. This allows the group members to orient the therapist.

When the therapist enters a partially gathered group, there is no way to know who has not been spontaneously involved in the process. The therapist, as the group's uniting factor, must gather all members by making verbal contact with each. This helps prevent the development of a schism between group members that may continue through the session and beyond.

Group members will repeat the gathering process to include late arrivals. The physical and visual interruptions of someone entering must be dealt with by acknowledging the person and orienting to them before the group can return its attention to the agenda (Pryor, 1984).

The primary function of the therapist during this segment is to visually and verbally establish contacts between members. The initial connecting factor among group members, their relationships with the therapist, will be generalized to the group through the actions of the therapist. Even groups that have been together for an extended time benefit from the therapist joining them at the gathering place, physically entering the conversational space, and making direct contact with each member. These actions serve to reaffirm the relationships within the group (Yalom, 1983).

Grouping

The formal beginning of the group should be the same at each session (Ely, 1985) and involve all group members. This segment reinforces the predictability of the group, thereby increasing the members' sense of safety.

A formal group government is utilized in this segment. Member leaders allow for the sharing of responsibility between members and the therapist, formally recognizes the abilities of those elected, and reduces challenges of the group leader by informal leaders (Shepherd, 1964). It also makes decision making a safer process and promotes the acceptance of personal and group responsibility (Yalom, 1983).

Business conducted during this segment includes the introduction of new members. There may be a set welcoming committee, or a member may be selected for this task. Formal role call is conducted to ensure participation by all members, reinforce personal identity, and orient members to each other (Yalom, 1983). The absence of members is made apparent and members' integration of the concept of object constancy is enhanced.

The final act of this business phase is the fine tuning of the plans for the main activity of the session. This includes reviewing the plan and making revisions to accommodate for absent members, unavailable supplies, and numerous other last minute details (Ely, 1985).

Throughout this segment of the session, the therapist provides guidance as the group makes the decisions (Yalom, 1983). The therapist helps the group problem solve rather than rescue members from cooperative decision making by providing solutions. The completion of this phase leads directly to the task.

Task

This is the action segment of the group. It is often the activity planned for this time that entices members to attend (Simons, 1985). There are three requirements that a task must meet to be used. First, the task must be experiential. It must also be useful to members in their daily lives (Ely, 1985). Lastly, it must be accomplishable within the time frame and physical restraints of the group (Yalom, 1983).

The goal of this segment is success (Fountain House, 1985). Tasks are designed so that each member can make a contribution to the end result. The large task is partialized into parts that individuals or small groups can complete. Competition should be avoided as it detracts from the underlying concept of group support and reliance (Ely, 1985).

Numerous activities lend themselves to groups. In the area of daily living skills, cooking, shopping, cleaning a member's apartment, writing a newsletter, and picking up litter in the park are examples that only touch on the possibilities. Movies, picnics, team sports, and window shopping are some of the appropriate leisure activities available in most areas.

Participation of individuals is not required during this segment. Contributions are encouraged (Fountain House, 1985). The ability of the member to contribute is repeatedly reinforced through recognition of the member's presence, requests for assistance, and encouragement to join in. The expected behaviors are visually demonstrated to members by the therapist's active involvement in the task completion.

The therapist does not release members from difficult situations. Instead, the therapist assists members to jointly problem solve, adapt the task, or enlist the assistance of another member. The therapist constantly monitors individual affect and behaviors, group mood, and safety factors. Members are assisted to become consciously aware of their internal responses to physical closeness, high activity levels, and other inherent aspects of the group (Pepper, Rylewicz, & Kirshner, 1982). Brief periods away from task are used to manage concentration impairments and frustrations.

Process

Recognition and integration are the objectives of this segment. The therapist helps members make an intellectual connection with what they have accomplished. This is done by verbally reviewing the difficulties and successes that members experienced (Yalom, 1983). The correlation between component tasks successfully completed and the final product is directly stated. Observed behaviors are verbally related to internal sensations which are, in turn, related to environmental stressors the members experienced during the task.

To the uninitiated observer, this segment may appear more like socialization than treatment. The Occupational Therapist, however, recognizes that treatment does not have to be formally constrained to be effective and purposefully elects an informal mode during this time. Spontaneous interaction among members not only provides important member opinions and ideas, it stimulates acceptable patterns of relating to others. These acceptable patterns are modeled by the therapist in the course of keeping the conversation on track (Yalom, 1983).

Planning

Having successfully completed one task, the group is prepared to plan for another. Planning is done in as much detail as possible. The therapist informs the group of the parameters (budget, supplies, location, space, time) within which the activity must occur, provides any desired visual aides (blackboard or large paper), and encourages the planning process (Ely, 1985).

Member-leaders solicit suggestions and lead the discussion about each proposal. The therapist points out salient factors that affect the feasibility of certain activities if the group does not. Some tasks will require preparation during one group session and completion in the next. Each member casts a vote for their preference of the options. This promotes the sense of individual effectance and control. The group and therapist then work together to identify the component parts of the task, and everyone present volunteers for the part they would like to work on.

This activity serves to reinforce the members' connections to each other (Pepper, Rylewicz, & Kirshner, 1982). It elicits commitments to participate and attend future groups. It also provides a concrete time reference and facilitates cognitive planning.

The final aspect of planning is the reiteration of the time, location, and main task of the next session. With this, the planning is finished and the group session is over. As members depart, the therapist should make direct contact with each, reaffirming the continuing relationship, individual contributions, and the expectation that the member will attend the next session.

VALUE OF OCCUPATIONAL THERAPY

The knowledge and skill of the Occupational Therapist are invaluable assets in activity focused group therapy of the type described. Applied theories and techniques of Occupational Therapy are what enable groups such as this to be an effective treatment modality.

The most obvious contribution is in the area of activity programming. The planning process can be guided by the therapist toward those tasks which address the holistic needs of the individual group members. The fact that the therapist's guidance and decisions are based in scientific knowledge is of key import. It is this process that makes the chosen activities prescriptive for the group rather than descriptive of the group.

The ability to separate activities into their basic component parts which can be successfully performed is another asset. More important, however, is the therapist's ability to observe an individual member at a task and immediately adapt the task to remediate or accommodate for the unique characteristics of the individual.

In this manner, the Occupational Therapist is an important member of both the treatment and diagnostic teams. Observations of the therapist may lead to a needed consultation/evaluation of conditions that may have gone unnoticed by other disciplines.

During the process segment of the group, the therapist can immediately provide members with specific information. Drawing from a broad knowledge base, the Occupational Therapist is prepared to explain how an activity is helpful to the many different internal systems of the member's body. The relationship between those systems and the individual's ability to function in certain situations can be clearly and simply described.

CONCLUSION

The group format and process described in this article demonstrates the vital role that Occupational Therapy plays in the effective group treatment of the chronically mentally ill. The ability to utilize scientifically based activity to address the many pressing needs of group members is a skill unique to assertively demonstrate this contribution to the field of mental health by continuing to develop and conduct groups which enable the chronically mentally ill members to develop socially acceptable behaviors and live safely within the community.

REFERENCES

Crabtree, L. H. (1984). Disability in young adult chronic patients at discharge from a private psychiatric hospital. *New Directions for Mental Health Services, 21*, 37-47.

Ely, A. R. (1985). Long-term group treatment for young 'schizopaths'. *Social Work, 30*(1), 5-10.

Fountain House. (1985). Unpublished training in the development and implementation of the Clubhouse model of treatment. *Fountain House*. New York.

Pepper, B. & Rylewicz, H. (1984). Treating the young male chronic patient: An update. *New Directions for Mental Health Services, 21*, 5-16.

Pepper, B., Rylewicz, H., & Kirshner, M. (1982). The uninstitutionalized generation: A new breed of psychiatric patient. *New Directions for Mental Health Services, 14*, 3-14.

Pryor, K. (1984). *Don't Shoot the Dog*. New York: Bantam.

Shepherd, C. R. (1964). *Small Groups: Some Sociological Perspectives*. Scranton: Chandler Publishing.

Simons, R. L. (1985). Inducement as an approach to exercising influence. *Social Work, 30*(1), 56-62.

Yalom, I. D. (1983). *Inpatient Group Psychotherapy*. New York: Basic Books.

Structured Craft Group Activities for Adolescent Delinquent Girls

Joyce Hardison, MS, OTR
Lela A. Llorens, PhD, OTR, FAOTA

SUMMARY. This was a study of the effects of a craft group for teenage delinquent girls with suspected vestibular processing difficulties. The craft group was led by an occupational therapist which met for two hour sessions lasting six weeks. There were 6 qualified participants, but only 3 were available as subjects for the study due to attrition prior to the pretest. Subjects were administered the Occupational Therapy Clinical Observation Evaluation, Bay Area Functional Performance Evaluation, and the King-Devick Saccadic Test for pre- and posttesting. Careful analysis of the craft group process and design indicated growth individually and collectively.

Joyce Hardison, Independent Contractor, 176 Camino Pablo, Orinda, CA 94563.

Lela A. Llorens, Professor, Chair and Graduate Coordinator, San Jose State University, San Jose, CA 95121.

The assistance of the following people is gratefully acknowledged: Marti Southam, MA, OTR; Bert Norcross, PhD; Kris Vensand, OTR; Nelson Clark, MS, OTR; Harley Baker, and Nancy Pulpaneck, MS, OTR. Thanks also to Arbutus Youth Association, Inc. and Palomares Group Homes for use of their facilities.

Note to the Reader: In the original study, from which this paper was abstracted, the group described herein was compared to a group that received a self-administered, therapist-supervised intervention. The sample was small and the design was flawed; however, because of the unexpected results that occurred with the group that employed crafts as the medium with therapist supervision, a decision was made to report these findings as a descriptive paper. The result of the study reporting the findings from both groups in detail is available from San Jose State University, "A Comparative Study of Group and Supervised Self-Administered Occupational Therapy with Female Adolescent Delinquents" by Joyce Hardison.

101

INTRODUCTION

Crafts is an area rarely examined by today's occupational therapists. However, it was discovered through research for an occupational therapy thesis that craft activities offered multiple benefits for a selected population of teenage delinquent girls. This information was gathered through a craft group, initially developed as a control group, of teenage delinquent girls, ages 16-18.

Occupational therapy is concerned with the quality of the individual's performance in activities of his or her daily life. It is the purpose of occupational therapy to prevent dysfunction, maintain function, and enhance the individual's functional ability in the area(s) of existing weakness so that maximum fulfillment in life roles and tasks (areas of occupational performance) may be experienced. Those areas include work, play/leisure and self-care activities. The skill areas (occupational performance components) of life roles and tasks are: Sensory integrative, motor, cognitive, psychological, and social. When performance skills are limited in any of the above areas, the individual's ability to meet daily life tasks is unsatisfactorily met, quantitatively and qualitatively.

In occupational therapy, choosing an appropriate and purposeful activity is considered essential for therapeutic change to occur or continue. Activities selected for therapeutic value must provide action, allow for repetition, and permit gradation. Hopkins, Smith and Tiffany (1978) reported that,

> The activities with which occupational therapy is primarily concerned are those which help to promote competence and achievement in the patient's or client's ability to function in her/his world. The three categories of self-care, work, and play, and the maintenance of a healthy balance in the individual's activity life, are an important focus of occupational therapy. (p. 118)

Occupational therapy uniquely approaches the person as a whole. Treatment is provided with the belief that deficit or dysfunctioning parts affect the whole and must be considered both in terms of parts and of the whole. The occupational performance components are considered the parts that make up the whole, as they include sensory integrative, motor, cognitive, psychological and social skill areas. If problems should arise from birth or later in life, thus inhibiting growth and development in any of the above areas, ultimately affecting life roles and tasks, then the functional potential of the individual could be limited. The value of human life and normal development are strong considerations when implementing a plan of intervention to encourage healthy development to occur or to continue. Two developmental theorists that promote this kind of intervention are Llorens and Reilly, both occupational therapists, researchers, and educators.

In describing a theory of Facilitating Growth and Development, Llorens proposed that,

> Occupational therapists focus on physical, social, and psychological parameters of human tasks and relationships. Within this context the therapist looks at individual functions and their integration, both during specific periods of life (horizontal development) and over the course of time (longitudinal development). The therapist's role is conceptualized as that of a change agent, facilitating the growth and development of the individual. (Clark and Allen, 1985, p. 39)

This theory is of special importance to the occupational therapist when considering therapeutic forms of intervention for adolescent juvenile delinquents.

In the Theory of Play, Reilly proposes that play is a specific component to learning. She believes that without play, learning would be thwarted and development of the person as a whole would be delayed. Utilizing general systems theory, she saw play as a part of the behavior system. She developed this assumption further by stating that, "Play is a subsystem of the imagination system of learning. The subsystems within play are exploratory, competency, and achievement behaviors" (Clark and Allen, 1985, p. 37).

According to the occupational performance frame of reference, the area of play/leisure, considered one of life's roles and tasks, included the use of crafts. Traditionally, craft activities were used in occupational therapy to improve quality of life, while occupying an individual's time, thereby promoting balance in the individual's life tasks of work, play/leisure and self-care.

DESCRIPTION OF THE CRAFT GROUP

Following is a discussion of how the research commenced. Six adolescent juvenile delinquent girls, ages 16-18, constituted the sample. These subjects were on probation for delinquent behavior, and were court appointed to reside in group homes, located in the greater San Jose area of California. These subjects were selected from two different group homes. Subjects from one group home became the experimental group, and subjects from the other, the control group, with three subjects in each group.

Subjects were administered the Occupational Therapy Clinical Observation Evaluation (OTCOE), Bay Area Functional Performance Evaluation (BaFPE), and the King-Devick Saccadic Test (K-D Saccadic) for pretesting and posttesting. It was determined after pretesting that all six subjects had vestibular processing difficulties, demonstrating slight to moderate impairment, although not conclusive due to the limitation of test materials.

The craft group, initially known as the control group, is the focus of this paper, and following is a description of the craft group. Three case studies are included to illustrate the kinds of benefits experienced by this group, and to illustrate the kinds of growth patterns that took place for each participant during the craft group, thereby demonstrating the strength of the craft group process and its design.

Mandatory participation by each member was implemented by the group home counselors to ensure group participation. All of the girls in the group home were involved in the group, while individual case studies involved only three of the girls, so the group size varied from 4-6 depending on how many of the girls were currently living in the home. The sessions were two hours long and lasted for six weeks. Crafts could be completed in 1-2 sessions and were selected and purchased by the researcher. They were also selected as age appropriate tasks for teenage girls as seen by the researcher. Craft activities varied in complexity, and included decoupage; macrame; molding, firing and painting clay/dough art projects made by the subjects; painting and dying Easter eggs; making sachets using potpourri; and selecting and painting small preformed ceramic magnets and lapel pins.

At the beginning of intervention, the subjects appeared interested in the activities, but soon became competitive and argumentative with each other. The subjects also became hesitant to participate wholeheartedly in some of the earlier projects, such as the macrame and the free-form dough art. Yet, they eagerly participated in decoupage, dying Easter eggs, making sachets and painting of small preformed ceramic lapel pins and magnets. While participating in these activities, the subjects began to cooperate with each other and interact in socially acceptable ways. These results were unexpected, but a pleasant surprise to the researcher. By the end of therapy, the subjects stated that they hated to see the group come to an end. They all seemed to enjoy the group, each other and the craft activities.

When analyzing the craft projects, those activities that have a low risk factor such as dying Easter eggs and painting preformed ceramic lapel pins and magnets, appeared to be enjoyed more by the subjects than activities that required more creativity, imagination, and fine motor skill and coordination. Macrame and free-form clay/dough art projects seemed to be intimidating to the subjects, probably because they offered less structure and required more imagination and experimentation with the material.

The group format took shape as parallel play, according to Mosey's five levels of group development. Mosey (1970) reported that, "Five types of developmental groups have been identified: Parallel, project, egocentric-cooperative, cooperative and mature" (p. 272). The activities were selected for the subject's enjoyment requiring few choices from the group. The researcher was responsible to see that each subject completed her tasks, and provided emotional support to each group member. None of the craft activities required joint effort; each project was designed for individual task completion. Towards the end of the treatment period, the group began to engage in project play, the second in Mosey's levels of group development. They began to cooperate and seek out suggestions and feedback from other members, and interacted positively with each other. This demonstrated growth and development individually and collectively.

This was illustrated by the way that the girls began to take risks in the group. Towards the end of therapy, they started exploring and experimenting with their craft projects. According to Reilly (1985), a person cannot proceed in developing advanced play behavior until the environment is considered safe and pleasurable. When basic needs for security are met then exploration of objects and the environment can commence. Satisfactory exploration leads to competency, and later to achievement behavior (Clark and Allen, p. 38). This kind of development would suggest the importance of the researcher as a therapeutic agent for change. It would also support the beliefs of Reilly, Mosey, Llorens, and Fidler, that play, via craft activities, is instrumental in promoting change in the areas of occupational performance (Clark and Allen, 1985; Mosey, 1970; and Fidler, 1981).

The design of the craft group provided nurturing from an adult figure; parallel play; opportunity for exploration, competency and achievement of craft projects; social stimulation and acceptance from peers. When comparing these aspects to the areas of occupational performance, every area was stimulated — sensorially, motorically, cognitively, psychologically, and socially, and thus learning and behavior were enhanced.

Sensorially they were stimulated through their systems of touch, sight and smells of differing projects. Each project required the use of fine and gross motor skills for task participation and completion. Cognitively they had to problem solve some of the tasks, and evaluate whether what they were doing met with their sense of completion, before going on to another project. As a result of this, they experienced heightened self-esteem through participation and completion of their projects, as noted by their growing enthusiasm for the group. Socially they were enhanced by the dynamics of group process as they grew individually and collectively from parallel to project play according to Mosey's levels of group development. It was concluded by the researcher that the changes noted on their posttest results could be attributed to a combination of the parallel play group design, the variety of craft activities, and the therapeutic value of the researcher as facilitator of the group. Following is a discussion of the three subjects as they experienced the group to better understand the dynamics of this group design.

Subject One, Larue, aged 16, demonstrated moderate vestibular processing difficulties on the pretest and mild-moderate vestibular processing difficulties on the posttest, with possible signs of organicity, noted on the posttest Draw A Person Test (see Tables 1, 2 and 3).

At the beginning of the group, Larue only observed with curiosity, and required encouragement to participate in the craft activities. She also stayed very close to the group home counselor and often demonstrated the "clingy" behavior of a young child. As the group continued; however, she demonstrated enthusiasm for the projects, and more mature social interaction with her peers as well. At the last session, she seemed very disappointed that the group had come to an end.

Following is a description of Larue's participation in the group. The first activity was decoupage. The researcher supplied magazines from which to cut pretty pictures to decoupage onto wood. However, Larue preferred to decoupage pictures of friends. By the end of the session, she appeared happy and was interacting with her peers, not clinging as much to the adults. The following week, free-form clay projects were introduced. Larue's design was a very simple heart. The following week, she painted the heart red with the counselor's name on it. She then gave it to her counselor, because she stated that she hoped it would make the counselor feel happy, since she thought the counselor seemed depressed. The counselor then reported to Larue that the heart made her feel better. The third session involved macrame projects, with choices to either make a key ring or hair decoration piece. Larue chose to make a key ring. This was a very difficult project for her. This task required ability to follow directions, motor plan, and demonstrate fine motor coordination. Due to the severity of her vestibular processing problems which contributed to these areas of functioning, she had great difficulty with this project. She showed no signs of difficulty with the next project; however, she enthusiastically participated in dying and painting of Easter eggs. She experimented with every color possible until she ended up with black eggs, and appeared very happy despite peer disapproval. When making sachets, Larue simply cut the

Table 1

Standing Balance Eyes Open and Closed

	Larue				Beth				Maria			
	Pretest		Posttest		Pretest		Posttest		Pretest		Posttest	
	^{a}R	^{b}L	R	L	R	L	R	L	R	L	R	L
a) Eyes Open	50	7.5	34	7.5	25	49	112	27	39	5	54.5	56
b) Eyes Closed	1.5	1	1.5	5	3	5	3	5	2.5	4	2.5	2

Note: ^{a}R = Right

   ^{b}L = Left

   ^{c}Numbers = Seconds

   No norms for this age group

Table 2

Occupational Therapy Clinical Observation Evaluation Results

	EXPERIMENTAL GROUP						CONTROL GROUP					
	Kim		Elizabeth		Kathy		Larue		Beth		Maria	
	[a]Pre	[b]Post	Pre	Post	Pre	Post	Pre	Post	Pre	Post	Pre	Post
Prone Extension	2	2	3	3	3	3	1	1	3	3	3	3
Cocontraction												
a) Arms/Trunk	2	2	2	3	1	2	1	1	[c]N.T.	N.T.	1	1
b) Neck	2	2	3	3	3	3	3	3	N.T.	N.T.	3	3
Supine Flexion	3	N.T.	3	1	2	2	1	1	3	3	1	3
Visual Pursuits												
a) In General	3	3	3	3	3	2	3	3	3	3	3	3
b) Across Midline	2	2	3	3	3	2	3	3	2	3	3	3
c) Quick Localization	2	2	3	3	3	3	3	3	2	2	3	3
d) Convergence	3	3	3	2	2	2	3	3	2	3	1	2
Preference												
a) Eye	R	R	L	R	R	R	R	R	R	R	R	R
b) Hand	L	L	L	R	R	R	R	R	R	R	R	R
Schilder's Arm Extension												
a) Choreoathetosis	2	3	3	3	2	2	2	3	3	3	2	3
b) Postural Changes												
1) Arms/Trunk	2	3	3	3	2	2	2	3	3	3	2	3
2) Head Resists	3	3	3	3	3	2	2	3	3	3	3	3
Assymetrical Tonic Neck Reflex												
a) Quadrupedal LUE	3	3	3	3	3	3	2	2	3	3	2	3
b) Quadrupedal RUE	3	3	3	3	3	3	3	3	3	3	2	3

Note: [a]Pre = Pretest
[b]Post = Posttest
[c]N.T. = Not tested
3 = Normal
2 = Having difficulty
1 = Inability to perform task
No norms for this age group

Table 3

Bay Area Functional Performance Evaluation Results

	Larue		Beth		Maria	
	[a]Pr [b]Pt		Pr	Pt	Pr	Pt
Sorting Shells	42	42	42	43	42	42
Bank Deposit	40	41	39	44	35	38
Draw A Floor Plan	31	38	40	43	33	37
Block Design	40	40	41	43	32	38
Draw A Person	40	37	42	42	36	40
TOTAL	211	215	222	233	193	210
Percent Change	↑.02		↑.05		↑.07	

Note: Task Points Possible = 44

Total Points Possible = 240

[a]Pr = Pretest

[b]Pt = Posttest

material, added the potpourri and tied a piece of yarn around it. She also appeared pleased with the end product. The last project was painting preformed ceramic magnets. She chose a rainbow. She used all of the possible colors when painting it and then covered it up with black. When asked why she did that, she said she did not know, but said that all of the other colors were underneath the black. She then proceeded to drop colors over it, making a "mess," with paint all over herself and the area in which she was painting.

The structure of the weekly meetings was very helpful for Larue. It provided her with an opportunity to explore and experiment with various kinds of textures and objects. She experienced immediate satisfaction with a variety of end products. She also received peer attention in a socially acceptable way, while given the chance to play as a child under the guidance of a nurturing adult. This also provided her with the opportunity to explore possible interests that could later develop into hobbies. It gave her an opportunity to grow in a creative but structured environment that appeared to enhance her self-image and esteem. Evidence of enhanced self-image was seen by the many risks she began to take, while demonstrating pleasure in each activity. Her human figure drawing, taken from the BaFPE, demonstrated increased signs of trust that had occurred on an unconscious level. The researcher concluded that compensatory mechanisms were reduced, as her posttest drawing was very bizarre, demonstrating possible organic problems that were not evident in the pretest drawing. Her defense mechanisms had probably lessened to the point where her true neuropsychological self could safely appear. The drawing also displayed vestibular processing problems due to the figure's unusual looking features and simple form.

Larue demonstrated neurological improvement on the Schilder's Arm Extension Test (Table 4), where she increased from a score of 2 to 3. She also scored a 2% increase on the BaFPE, with an overall score of 211 on the pretest to 215 on the posttest.

In general, the researcher concluded that Larue had made unexpected gains because of the structure and variety of play that was offered to her in the weekly craft group. This group encouraged change that affected her vestibular system, as the activities involved her tactile, visual, gustatory, proprioceptive, auditory, limbic, and vestibular systems. The craft group encouraged developmental growth to occur, that was evidenced by her posttest results, and heightened social behavior in the group.

Subject Two, Beth, aged 16, demonstrated mild vestibular processing difficulties noted by her pretest and posttest human figure drawings (Table 3). The O.T. Clinical Observation Evaluation demonstrated problem areas in Visual Pursuit and Standing Balance with Eyes Closed (Tables 1 and 2). However, Standing Balance with Eyes Closed did not change on the posttest, but remained a problem, which supports evidence of a continued vestibular processing dysfunction.

The following is a description of her experiences in the craft

Table 4

King-Devick Saccadic Test

	Larue		Beth		Maria	
	^{a}Pre	^{b}Post	Pre	Post	Pre	Post
Test 1	26	29	19	16	17	15.05
Test 2	27	28.05	22.05	18	17	12.04
Test 3	22	30	21	20.08	17.07	16.08

Note: ^{a}Pre = Pretest

^{b}Post = Posttest

Numbers = Seconds (test completion time)

No norms for this age group

group that expressed the changes that occurred. In the first session, Beth, too, chose pictures of friends and family to decoupage versus pictures of scenery. It appeared to the researcher that this may have been an attempt to make their special relationships permanent, by placing their pictures on wood. The next week, she was unable to participate because of a drinking violation that placed her in Juvenile Hall. The third week, she refused to participate in macrame, but sat with the group throughout the entire session giving disruptive comments that required limit-setting by the researcher. Unfortunately, Beth was allowed to take a date night the following week by prearranged approval from the counselor, unknown to the researcher.

It was not until the fifth session that Beth again participated in the group. She demonstrated creativity in the use of materials when making sachets. She made pom-poms of the yarn then tied them around the sachets. She also encouraged other girls to follow her example. It appeared that she was having a very good time. During the last session, she selected a rainbow and ice cream cone to paint. She demonstrated good use of colors, and seemed to enjoy the activity. However, in the beginning of the session, she became competitive and sarcastic with other group members, belittling their projects. When confronted by the researcher, she quickly settled down, and became a supportive member of the group. The researcher felt that Beth needed to test limits for inner control and adult attention, as she immediately calmed down following the confrontation.

Her drawings illustrated and supported the changes in behavior that were noted in the group. Her posttest human figure drawing displayed signs of organic problems evidenced by the structure and quality of drawing. The researcher believes that her true neuropsychological self became apparent in the posttest drawing, due to the design of the craft group, as previously described.

Her drawing of a floorplan was very exacting, but off center to the right on the pretest. While the posttest drawing was in the middle of the paper, and was not completed with the exactness that was demonstrated in the pretest. However, the rooms though messier in line quality had doors, while the pretest had no doorways to other rooms or to the outside. These drawings also demonstrated problems with spatial relationships and motor planning, as there was considerable empty space between rooms that was unidentified. The floorplan drawings support the human figure drawings as they demonstrate that her level of trust had increased, allowing for more accurate feelings to appear, demonstrating increased vestibular processing to emerge.

The craft group was very beneficial for Beth as she made gains in the area of Visual Pursuit (Table 2). Her scores of 2 in Crossing Midline and Eye Convergence improved to a normal score of 3, with an existing problem noted only in Quick Localization. Improved Visual Pursuit was also seen on the K-D Saccadic posttest (Table 4). She made tremendous gains on the BaFPE (Table 3). Her overall score increased 5% with scores of 222 to 233 on the posttest.

Her improved performance was believed to be, in part, a result of the structure of the craft group. It provided exploratory play with an end-product as an immediate reward while under the guidance of a nurturing adult. The craft activities helped to simulate the tactile, visual, gustatory, auditory, limbic, proprioceptive and vestibular systems. This kind of group offered Beth the opportunity to take risks, explore and develop possible interests with nurturing, but firm support from an adult. At the same time, her level of trust increased to a level that allowed a more accurate picture of her neuropsychological self to safely appear, as evidenced in the human figure posttest drawing.

The researcher made the assumption that she had vestibular processing difficulties as evidenced by the human figure and floorplan drawings, both pretest and posttest. This group offered Beth a chance to grow and develop neuropsychologically in such a way that her behavior was positively affected. This may have been specifically due to the design of the craft group.

Subject Three, Maria, 16 years of age, displayed mild-moderate vestibular processing difficulties on the pretest to mild difficulties on the posttest (Table 2). It was determined that she had vestibular processing problems because of her pretest results in the O.T. Clinical Observation Evaluation and the BaFPE drawings (Table 3).

Her scores are worth reviewing as she improved in every area but Standing Balance with Eyes Closed (Table 1). Maria had demonstrated great difficulty in several areas of the O.T. Clinical Observation pretest evaluation that improved on the posttest. She had only attained a 1 on cocontraction of the Arms and Trunk, Supine Flexion, and Eye Convergence. On the posttest, she attained a normal score of 3, except for a 2 on Eye Convergence. She also improved on the Schilder's Arm Extension Test and Asymmetrical Tonic Neck Reflex Test (Table 4) where she increased from scores of 2 to normal scores of 3. She even improved on Standing Balance with Eyes Open, demonstrating better sensory integration because of her similar posttest times. She increased from 39 right (R) and 5 Left (L) seconds to 54.5 (R) and 56 (L) seconds on the posttest. She also made considerable gain on the K-D Saccadic test and the BaFPE. Her overall score improved 7% with scores of 193 on the pretest to 210 on the posttest. The K-D Saccadic test scores improved from 17, 17, and 17.05 seconds to 15.05, 12.04, and 16.08 seconds on the posttest. Reasons for such an astounding improvement will be discussed following a description of her group activities.

The craft group was extremely beneficial for Maria as evidenced by her posttest results. Maria participated with enthusiasm as the group began. She, like the other group members, chose pictures of family members to decoupage. For the same reasons, the researcher suggests that she, too, was attempting to hold onto the value of those relationships by decoupaging their pictures onto wood, to be forever treasured. The following week Maria did not attend the group, because she too, was in Juvenile Hall for breaking a drinking rule. The following week she, like Beth, did not participate in the group, only observed, probably due to Beth's influence. However, from the following week to the end she participated with great fervor.

Maria did not participate in dying of Easter eggs. She created dough art, the activity from the previous week, which she requested and was permitted to do. When making sachets the next week, Maria copied the design that Beth suggested to her, using pom-poms for bows to tie around the sachets. She seemed to enjoy the project, as she was very talkative and verbally supportive of other group members and their work. In the fifth group meeting, the group home counselor mentioned to the researcher that Maria had joined a gym, and seemed a lot happier since the group's commencement. During the last project, she selected two ceramic figures, a mouse and a rainbow. She seemed to require a lot of support as she often asked for the researcher's approval of her work. She seemed easily distracted, while busily interacting socially with the other group members.

Maria probably made tremendous gains because of the group structure and activities that were offered to her in combination with her vestibular stimulation activities at the gym, where she attended regularly. Her drawings also suggested that more trust had occurred, probably because of the group's design.

These results were further illustrated on the BaFPE drawings. On the pretest human figure drawing, she had refused to draw a figure below the head, and had erased a very large rounded mouth for another mouth that was not quite as large. This demonstrated strong signs of avoidance and dependency needs. On the posttest, she had drawn a person crying with a body that lacked feet and arms. This was significant to the researcher because she appeared very jovial and affectionate during the posttest evaluation, so her drawing of a person crying was a surprise. The researcher believes that this was probably a picture of her true self, with many fears, confusing thoughts, and much sadness due to past experiences in combination with vestibular processing difficulties. In general, the group was very influential in providing an arena for exploration, discovery, and change for Maria, with the confines of play activities with a nurturing adult figure that provided her with a healthy foundation to grow and develop further.

IMPLICATIONS FOR PRACTICE

Only modest implications can be drawn from this study given the sample size; however, the results suggest that occupational therapists can be effective in the use of craft groups when working with adolescents who have problems of delinquency and vestibular processing. With further evidence, early childhood education may be the vehicle of choice to introduce more purposeful play, along with academic learning in the primary grades, to enhance sensory perception, motor coordination, and cognitive, psychological, and social ability.

RECOMMENDATIONS FOR FUTURE RESEARCH

To continue this research and to better control for researcher bias, the design should be structured so that one therapist tests the subjects and another supervises and leads treatment. To validate the effectiveness of this design, subjects in this study should be tested 3 to 6 months following cessation of treatment to determine if there are lasting effects. Further study of the human figure drawing for possible use as a screening tool for vestibular processing seems warranted.

CONCLUSIONS

The purpose of this study is to illustrate the strengths and design of a craft group with teenage delinquent girls, ages 16-18. The individuals of this group experienced changes in all five areas of occupational performance; sensory-integration, motor, cognitive, psychological, and social. It was concluded that improvement could be attributed to its design: Nurturing adult figure (therapist); parallel play; and fine motor activities that promoted exploration and experimentation.

REFERENCES

Clark, P. N. and Allen, A. S. (1985). *Occupational Therapy For Children*. Missouri: C. V. Mosby Co.
Fidler, G. S. (1981). From crafts to competence. *American Journal of Occupational Therapy, 35* (9), 567-573.
Hopkins, H. L. and Smith, H. D. (Eds.) (1978). *Willard and Spackman's Occupational Therapy* (5th ed.). Charles B. Slack Inc.
Mosey, A. C. (1970). The concept and use of developmental groups. *American Journal of Occupational Therapy, 24* (4), 272-275.

Concept and Use
of The Social Skills Game
to Facilitate Group Interaction:
A Case Study

Holly Harper Love, MA, OTR

SUMMARY. A primary goal of occupational therapy is to improve psychiatric patients' social interaction skills. The role of the therapist, in this effort, is to provide opportunities for patients to practice and learn more effective ways of relating with others. Theorists in the profession have encouraged occupational therapists to consider the use of group games to accomplish this objective.

Although the use of games has been reported by occupational therapists who work with mentally retarded children and adults, the use of games with psychiatric populations has received little attention in the literature.

This article describes the use of The Social Skills Game to facilitate social interaction and the development of social skills in a psychiatric population.

Holly Harper Love received her Master of Arts degree in occupational therapy from Tufts University-Boston School of Occupational Therapy. She has worked as an occupational therapist in acute psychiatry since the completion of her graduate training. She is currently Senior Occupational Therapist on the combined medical-psychiatric unit at Stanford University Hospital. Mailing address: PT/OT Department, Hoover Pavilion, Room N035, Stanford University Hospital, Stanford, CA 94305.

The author wishes to thank Margot C. Howe, EdD, OTR and Sharon L. Schwartzberg, EdD, OTR for their advice and inspiration during the development of The Social Skills Game; and Dawn Warrington, OTR, and Kathy Hanlan, OTR, for their assistance and support during the initial field testing of The Social Skills Game.

The Social Skills Game was copyrighted by the author. Inquiries regarding the availability of the game may be directed to the author.

119

INTRODUCTION

A common problem shared by most psychiatric patients seen in occupational therapy is one of inadequate social skills. This deficiency severely impairs an individual's ability to establish and maintain interpersonal relationships which are an essential part of human life (Argyle, 1969; Mosey, 1981).

Psychiatric occupational therapy, in its commitment to the promotion of skills required for adaptive and productive daily living, has directed much of its attention toward enhancing patients' social skills. The use of activity groups has been firmly established as a means to accomplish this objective (Schwartzberg, Howe, & McDermott, 1982). These groups are structured in such a way that will facilitate social interaction between group members and, therefore, provide opportunities for patients to practice and learn more effective social behaviors.

Group games were once considered to be an important occupational therapy activity for increasing social interaction among psychiatric patients, although they are not currently in widespread use (Kielhofner & Miyake, 1981). Games are consistent with the basic philosophy of occupational therapy and should be considered for clinical use (Huff, 1981; Kielhofner & Miyake, 1981). Games promote adaptive learning by providing a milieu which: (a) requires that the individual takes an active role in the process, (b) contains components and tasks which elicit the individual's adaptive responses, (c) focuses the individual's attention on the tasks of the game, thereby permitting the subconscious centers to integrate and organize learning and skills, and, (d) provides both intrinsic and extrinsic reward for successful mastery. These characteristics have been identified by King (1978) as the four characteristics of the adaptive process and the core of occupational therapy.

Hyde, York, and Wood (1948) proposed that "interest in games may be used to awaken social responses in patients otherwise apathetic and withdrawn or confused, agitated and deluded" (p. 304). These authors emphasized the need for more research concerning the use of games with adult psychiatric patients in order to better understand the association between game play and increased social interaction between the players. During the last several decades, this need for further research has not been actively addressed. The few studies which have been reported in the occupational therapy literature have focused on the use of games with developmentally delayed children (Huff, 1981) and mentally retarded adults (Kielhofner & Miyake, 1981; Nochajski & Gordon, 1987).

THE CONCEPT AND USE OF OCCUPATIONAL THERAPY ACTIVITY GROUPS

According to Mosey (1981), activity groups can provide: (a) a laboratory for living; a social microcosm which promotes learning by doing, (b) a setting similar to that found in the normal developmental process, (c) a degree of structure and organization, (d) an opportunity for constructive use of the nonhuman environment, (e) an opportunity to focus on the doing process, and (f) a tangible means of measuring the progress of each group member and the progress of the group as a whole. In short, the necessary components for the development of interpersonal skills that are required for effective functioning in the community (Mumford, 1974). It is important to note, however, that groups are not inherently therapeutic (Levine, 1979). For instance, Mosey (1973) wrote that a common problem in activity groups is that the patients tend to direct most of their communication to group leaders rather than to one another. When this occurs, the group loses much of its potential for learning. Groups must be structured in a way that is appropriate for the patients in the group in order to accomplish their particular objectives. Schwartzberg, Howe, and McDermott (1982) wrote that "unlike the first activity groups used in occupational therapy, the leadership, group and activity processes used today are structured and monitored in a more theoretical and systematic fashion to achieve the aim of improved social interaction skill" (p. 1). As they are currently used, activity groups are based on an integration of three theoretical systems: (1) the role of purposeful activities in the development and maintenance of skills needed for participation in society, (2) the study of the dynamics of small groups, and (3) identification of factors in small groups that can be manipulated to promote positive changes in group members; that is, the general therapeutic factors in small groups (Mosey, 1981). It is beyond the scope of this report to describe these theoretical systems, however, information relative to each will be presented as it applies to the use of group games in occupational therapy.

GAMES AS OCCUPATIONAL THERAPY TOOLS

Games have long been considered important and legitimate tools for occupational therapy (Hopkins & Smith, 1978). In 1922. Adolf Meyer stated that in treating psychiatric patients, "we naturally begin with a simple regime of pleasurable ease, the creation of an orderly rhythm in the atmosphere . . . perhaps with some music and restful dance and play" (p. 641). Play and games came to be recognized as a "critical dimension in the normal balance of daily life patterns" (Vandenberg & Kielhofner, 1982) for adults as well as children. Play is a form of learning by doing (Reilly, 1974). It is a manifestation of man's natural drive to action in the service of learning, exploration and discovery of himself and his environment (Fidler & Fidler, 1978). White (1971) wrote that man's inherent drive for active exploration and mastery of the environment should be understood as an urge to improve this competence in dealing with the environment. It has been suggested that learning which occurs during play is organized on a subcortical level (Ayres, 1973; King, 1978). During play, the individual's conscious attention is directed toward the play activity and the enjoyment it provides. The "fun component" of play permits almost subliminal learning; that is, learning without trying or being conscious of the learning process (Glazier, 1969). Vandenberg and Kielhofner (1982) proposed that it is not only what the individual learns in play that is important, but also how the player learns to adapt his behavior to external conditions in the environment. Play facilitates flexible behavior which prepares the individual to adapt his behavior to particular circumstances (Bruner, 1976). Game play adds a social component to play. Within the game context the individual develops a sense of himself in an organized social group (Mead, 1934). Players perform a set of responses and organize them in accordance to the rules of the game and the responses of others. Participation in games "will lead to making friends, getting along with others, learning to share, compete, cooperate, take turns, and a generally more satisfactory social adjustment" (Cartledge & Milburn, 1980, p. 204). Kielhofner and Miyake (1981) maintained that "in the game one learns to be social and to do social life" (p. 376). Reilly (1974) commented that games teach players the way in which social relationships are ordered by rules. She wrote, "man learns to act with confidence because he expects others to act in certain ways. He is able to respond to these ways of acting because the social interaction game has a form, a set of rules, which determines how the other must act toward us" (p. 108). Games provide a meaningful, risk-free milieu for active exploration of "real-life" experiences (Glazier, 1969; Reilly, 1974). Avedon and Sutton-Smith (1971) emphasized that in terms of the therapeutic value of game play, it is not the game played that is important, instead it is how the game helps players learn to relate to the other players.

Hyde, York, and Wood (1948) wrote that the prime function of games in occupational therapy is to improve the socialization of psychiatric patients. These investigators conducted a study to determine the effectiveness of simple games in improving the socialization of adult male psychiatric patients. A secondary component of the study was to determine the effectiveness of using hospital personnel to initiate the games on the wards. A series of forty-eight, fifteen-minute observations were made of all activities which took place in the patients' smoking room with no attempt to primarily observe game activities. A second series of observations were then made of special game activities initiated by ward personnel in order to determine their part in stimulating socialization. The games used during both observation series included jig-saw puzzles, checkers, Chinese Checkers, Monopoly, playing cards, and Cribbage. The results of this study revealed that: (a) although game activity took place without the presence of ward personnel, there was more social interaction between patients during games which included personnel, (b) the more participants there were in a game, the more the game attracted patients to observe and/or participate in the game, (c) the simpler, more commonplace games attracted less interest than the better implemented, more unusual games, and (d) when participants "played to the audience" with running comments about the game or interesting general conversation, more patients were attracted to the game. These investigators concluded that more research was needed in order to better understand the factors which promoted the fullest participation of patients in games. Little research has been reported in this area. One study, conducted by Conte, Otero, and Gladfelter (1961), attempted to objectively evaluate the effects of occupational therapy techniques and the development of interpersonal relationships on overall improvement of chronic schizophrenics. The study subjects were engaged in a program consisting of intensive occupational therapy described as reading, movies, activities of daily living, bus rides, cooking, games and calisthenics. The results of the study suggested that this program led to improvement in the patients' ability to relate to others. In another study, subjective observations of psychiatric patients in a Veterans Hospital revealed that playing the card game Bridge stimulated interest and social interaction among patients (Raymond, 1963). This researcher concluded that "not only has this program helped return patients to the community, but as a tool for recreation, it has boosted morale on the ward considerably" (p. 226).

Druckenbrod (1981) investigated the use of games as a therapeutic treatment approach for juvenile delinquent boys. Subjects were engaged in table games for one and one-half hours, two times per week for a period of five weeks. In conjunction with the games, subjects discussed the implications of obeying rules in games as well as in the community. The subjects took a story completion test which measured moral judgment, altruism and honesty, before and after the game program. The results of the study, although inconclusive, revealed that all subjects' scores on the test either improved or remained the same.

A review of more recent occupational therapy literature reveals a paucity of research concerning the use of games in psychiatric settings. Reported use of games has been limited to teaching mentally deficient children daily living skills (Hurff, 1981); improving the general physical, emotional, social and cognitive performance of mentally retarded adults (Kielhofner & Miyake, 1981); and, teaching community living skills to adults with developmental disabilities (Nochajski & Gordon, 1987). Hurff (1981) stressed that "games should be acknowledged as a medium for training the handicapped population, and occupational therapists should report their research, development and refinement of game techniques and the use of games as part of the therapeutic armamentarium" (p. 731, 733).

THE SOCIAL SKILLS GAME

The Social Skills Game (Love, 1982) was developed for use in an occupational therapy social skills group on an acute psychiatric unit for adult and adolescent in-patients. The purpose of the game was to provide group members with opportunities to practice and learn more effective ways of relating to others in socially stimulating, yet non-threatening milieu.

The game equipment consists of: a game board, four sets of "skill builder cards," Free Pass cards, the playing pieces, and one die. The game board is divided into four sections and the spaces on the board, in each of these sections, are associated with the social skills required for handling these four types of social situations. For example: in the "Meeting New People" section of the board, players are required to introduce themselves to other players and initiate informal conversations with other members of the group; in the "Getting What You Need with Words" section of the board, the players practice asking for assistance and/or advice; in the "Constructive Comments" section of the board, players practice giving and receiving compliments and constructive criticism; and, in the "Saying 'No' without Feeling Guilty" section of the board, players practice turning down unwanted invitations or advice, and requests made by others.

The game play procedures consist of taking turns rolling the die and moving ahead on the game board the appropriate number of spaces. Some spaces on the game board direct players to draw a particular type of game card. With the exception of the Free Pass cards, the game cards describe a social situation common to daily life either on the hospital ward or in the community. The desired outcome of the situation is also described on the game card. A player who draws a game card is asked to read the card out loud and then to select one or more other players to role play the situation with him. After the role playing, group members are encouraged to discuss the performance and offer feedback to the performers. Each player who contributes to the role play earns the number of points specified on the particular game card. The group may also decide to award points to players who provided feedback concerning the role play situation. Free Pass cards may be obtained by players who have accumulated fifteen points. These cards entitle a player to skip one turn if he does not wish to role play a certain situation described on a game card he has drawn.

The value of points is limited to obtaining Free Pass cards and determining the winner of the game if the game must be stopped before a player has reached the "Finish."

The Social Skills Game (henceforth, The Game), was designed to represent a synthesis of the criteria for purposeful activities proposed by Hopkins and Smith (1978). These criteria are:

1. *Be goal directed*; have some purpose or reason for their use. The overt goals of The Game are: (a) to be the first player to move through the game board spaces from "Start" to "Finish," (b) to practice and learn more effective ways of relating with other people, (c) to establish individual goals, on a self-evaluation questionnaire, and work toward accomplishing those goals, and (d) to have fun! The covert goals of the game are to: (a) promote verbal interaction between patients in the group, in progressively more difficult hypothetical situations, requiring increasingly higher levels of social skills, and (b) promote group cohesiveness and trust.

2. *Have some significance and usefulness to the individual in relation to his interests and roles*. Prior to playing The Game, the group leader(s) and group members discuss the importance of social skills and social interaction in daily life. This is done to clarify the significance of the skills learned through playing The Game.

3. *Require some level of mental or physical participation on the part of the individual*. The Game requires that the individual is physically present during game play and game play requires some level of verbal interaction between players.

4. *Be aimed toward prevention of malfunction and/or maintenance or improvement of function and quality of life*. The Game is aimed toward improvement of present social skills and prevention of further malfunction in this area which could be caused by lack of opportunities for structured and "safe" social experiences due to hospitalization and/or the effects of a mental illness. In light of the central role which human rela-

tionships play in one's life, any improvement of one's social skills will improve the quality of the individual's life.

5. *Reflect involvement in life tasks* such as activities of daily living, play and work, thereby increasing the individual's competencies required for performance in his occupational roles. The Game is a play activity in that participation in the game is intended to be fun and spontaneous. There is a work component as well, which entails discussing social skills deficits and establishing goals to improve one's skills. Social skills are important life skills, required for performance in one's occupational roles. Therefore, participation in The Game is intended to increase players' competency for performance in their occupational roles. Players are encouraged to discuss individual problems which relate directly to their various roles in and out of the hospital.

6. *Relate to the individual's interests.* The individual should be involved in choosing the activity. Patients choose to join the social skills group and to participate in The Game. In order to be of interest to the players, the game tasks are designed to reflect common social situations which occur on the hospital unit as well as in the community. Also, during game play, players are encouraged to discuss individual experiences or concerns which relate to the tasks of The Game.

7. *Be adaptable and gradable.* The Game may be adapted and graded to the individual needs and skills of the players in various ways: (a) the game tasks move from a parallel group level to the highest potential level of the group. For example, during the first two groups sessions, patients complete a self-evaluation questionnaire concerning their social skills and deficits; no social interaction is required on the part of the group members, although they are encouraged to interact and are supported by the group leader(s) to do so. As the game progresses, the game tasks gradually require more interaction, and (b) during each game play session, the group leader(s) encourage increasingly more interaction between players. For example, during the first several game play sessions, players receive social reinforcement for simply introducing themselves to another group member; later in The Game, the group

leader(s) will encourage players to interact more. The group
leader(s) grade each game task in accordance with individual
patient's capabilities and goals.
8. *Be determined through the occupational therapist's profes-*
sional judgment based on the profession's body of knowledge.
The Game was designed to incorporate the theoretical founda-
tions of the concept and use of purposeful activities and activity groups.

Role play and feedback are discussed in the literature as important components in the natural process of learning social skills (Argyle, 1969; Bruner, 1976; Mosey, 1973). Various investigators and
clinicians have developed social skill training programs based on
the use of these techniques (Goldstein, 1973, 1979; Hersen, Eisler,
& Miller, 1973; Liberman, King, DeRisi, & McCann, 1975). These
programs consist of a small group situation for direct training of
social skills. The training methods include role playing social situations that trainees find difficult in their everyday lives; modeling of
social behaviors by the group leader and other trainees to provide
information relative to alternate ways of handling social situations;
social reinforcement and feedback on the role played behavior; and,
specific homework assignments to be completed between training
sessions. According to Falloon (1981), important guidelines followed in the programs are that: (a) the emphasis is on behavior
change in real-life situations, not merely improved function in the
training group, (b) patients are encouraged to meet and help one
another with their homework tasks outside group meetings, (c) positive feedback is stressed during the group sessions, (d) the themes
of the sessions are frequently programmed by the therapist from
prior knowledge of the patient's specific difficulties with social interaction, and (e) treatment in time-limited; usually a three-month
program. The effectiveness of these training programs has been
documented for significant improvement in social skills (Falloon,
Lindley, McDonald, & Marks, 1977; Goldstein, 1979) as well as
the promotion of group cohesiveness and development (Falloon,
1981). Each of these studies emphasizes the importance of role
play, modeling and reinforcement in the success of the training program. Mosey (1973) wrote that role playing is an important exam-

ple of learning by doing. She mentioned the purpose of role playing
is either to gain better understanding of "real-life" situations or to
practice some new type of behavior, or both. Hughes and Mullins
(1981) have observed that psychiatric patients who were considered
to be withdrawn, have been active participants in role playing exercises. These authors recommend the use of role playing to promote
participation in the occupational therapy treatment process.

The role of the group leader is another important part of The
Social Skills Game. Otto (1979) proposed that the leader of a play
group should be a facilitator, resource person, consultant, observer
and listener. Kielhofner and Miyake (1981) provided four other
guidelines for leaders of game groups which expand upon Otto's
suggestions. These guidelines are intended to maximize the player's
game play behavior in an effort to actualize the full learning potential of the play experience. The guidelines are:

1. *Grade the complexity.* The complexity of the game tasks of
   The Game are graded within each game play session as well as
   over the series of game play sessions. The group leader(s) ac-
   complishes this by arranging the game cards in such a way that
   the least difficult game cards will be drawn by the players
   first, and the more difficult game cards will be drawn later in
   the game play session. Group leaders also provide increasingly more feedback for players following their role playing
   and may ask players more questions about the role playing as
   the game progresses.
2. *Level relationships.* The group leader(s) shares the role of
   "game player" with the other group members. The group
   leader(s) joins the players in playing The Game.
3. *Coach and model.* Throughout The Game, the group leader(s)
   offers constructive feedback (coaching) concerning the players' performance. The group leader(s) also serves as a role
   model for performing the game play tasks.
4. *Keep the game context and continuity.* The group leader(s)
   works to keep the game context by redirecting players' attention to the game when necessary. The group leader(s) also
   works to maintain a playful, fun group process as much as
   possible. More serious discussions, however, are an important

part of The Game and the group leader(s) should initiate and support such discussions when appropriate. The group leader(s) may also need to remind players of the game rules and the purpose of the game. If game play carries over to several group meetings, it may be helpful to remind patients where the game was stopped at the end of the previous session. When appropriate, the group leader(s) may encourage players to share parts of the leadership role.

FIELD TESTING OF
THE SOCIAL SKILLS GAME

The game was field tested on an acute psychiatric unit for adult and adolescent patients within a community hospital. Twelve patients, male and female, between the ages of nineteen and seventy-five years, all with the diagnosis of Major Depression, were recruited to join an occupational therapy social skills group. Criteria for admission to the group were that: (a) the patient could benefit from social skills training, and (b) the patient could tolerate a group situation which involved some degree of verbal interaction with others. Patients experiencing a psychotic episode were considered inappropriate for this activity. The primary activity of the group was playing The Social Skills Game. The group met for two fifty-minute sessions each week for a period of four weeks. Group attendance fluctuated from seven to twelve patients. The length of each session ranged from thirty-five to fifty minutes. The group was co-led by an occupational therapy intern and a Registered Occupational Therapist. A Registered Nurse also attended, and participated in game play.

The group sessions consisted of: (a) two "warm-up" sessions in which the group leaders and group members discussed the importance of social skills; the concept and use of role playing; and examples of goals that could be worked on in the group. All group members completed a self-evaluation questionnaire concerning their social skills, and then discussed their goals with the group, (b) five game play sessions during which the group played The Social Skills Game. Before and after playing, the group typically discussed the game and/or the progress of the group. The winner was determined at the end of the last game session, and (c) one termination session during which the group engaged in an informal discussion about The Game and individual progress in the group. Refreshments were served to reinforce the social component of this session.

Subjective observations of the group suggested that:

1. *Patients seemed to enjoy playing The Game.* This was reflected in the general tone of the group process which was consistently spontaneous, bright and engaged. Most patients in the group mentioned to the group leaders that they enjoyed The Game and that they looked forward to the group sessions.
2. *Patients seemed to interact with each other more often than with the group leaders.* This was particularly true when patients chose another individual in the group to perform a role play with them; patients typically chose other patients.
3. *There appeared to be a high level of cohesiveness in the group.* Few patients were absent from the group unless they had another commitment during the group meeting time. Patients seemed concerned about absent members, and often asked where the absent members were. Patients seemed to enjoy being a part of this group.
4. *Patients gained an increased awareness of their social skills* and of the importance of practicing them in hypothetical situations before encountering similar situations outside of the game context. One patient commented that he would like to role play a job interview; another patient mentioned that he would like to practice social skills related to dating.

Subsequent use of The Game with similar psychiatric populations has continued to support these findings.

CONCLUDING REMARKS

The value of game play in learning and adaptation is an important part of occupational therapy theory (Reilly, 1974; Robinson, 1977; Takata, 1971). Based on theoretical formulations, it has been recommended that occupational therapists consider the use of games to promote social skill development in clients (Hurff, 1981; Hyde,

York, & Wood, 1948; Kielhofner & Miyake, 1981). The Social Skills Game is an example of how a board game can be used to successfully apply occupational therapy theory relative to the therapeutic value of activity groups.

REFERENCES

Argyle, M. (1969). *Social interaction.* New York: Atherton Press.

Avedon, E., & Sutton-Smith, B. (1971). *The study of games.* New York: John Wiley & Sons, Inc.

Ayres, A. (1973). *Sensory integration and learning disorders.* Los Angeles: Western Psychological Services.

Bruner, J. (1976). Nature and uses of immaturity. In J. Bruner, A. Jolly, & K. Sylva (Eds.). *Play: Its role in development and evolution.* New York: Basic Books.

Cartledge, G., & Milburn, J. (Eds.) (1980). *Teaching social skills to children.* New York: Pergamon Press.

Conte, W., Otero, M., & Gladfelter, J. (1961). Effects of intensive occupational therapy on chronic schizophrenic patients. *American Journal of Occupational Therapy, 15*, 103-105, 128.

Druckenbrod, C. (1981). *Games: An occupational therapy treatment mode for juvenile delinquent boys.* Unpublished research paper, Medical College of Virginia.

Falloon, I. (1981). Interpersonal variables in behavioral group therapy. *British Journal of Medical Psychology, 54*, 133-141.

Falloon, I., Lindley, P., McDonald, R., & Marks, I. (1977). Social skills training of outpatient groups: A controlled study of rehearsal and homework. *British Journal of Psychiatry, 131*, 599-609.

Fidler, G., & Fidler, J. (1978). Doing and becoming: Purposeful activity and self-actualization. *American Journal of Occupational Therapy, 32*, 305-310.

Glazier, R. (1969). *How to design educational games.* Cambridge, Massachusetts: ABT Associates.

Goldstein, A. (1973). *Structured learning therapy: Toward a psychotherapy for the poor.* New York: Academic Press.

Goldstein, A. (1979). Structured learning therapy: Development and evaluation. *American Journal of Occupational Therapy, 33*, 635-639.

Hersen, M., Eisler, R., & Miller, R. (1973). Development of assertive responses: Clinical measurement and research considerations. *Behaviour Research and Therapy, 11*, 505-522.

Hopkins, H., & Smith, H. (Eds.) (1978). *Willard and Spackman's occupational therapy* (5th Ed.). Philadelphia: J.B. Lippincott Company.

Hughes, P., & Mullins, L. (1981). *Acute psychiatric care: An occupational therapy guide to exercises in daily living.* Thorofare, New Jersey: Charles B. Slack, Inc.

Hurff, J. (1981). A gaming technique: An assessment and training tool for individuals with learning deficits. *American Journal of Occupational Therapy, 35,* 728-735.

Hyde, R., York, R., & Wood, A. (1948). Effectiveness of games in a mental hospital. *Occupational Therapy and Rehabilitation, 27,* 304-308.

Kielhofner, G., & Miyake, S. (1981). The therapeutic use of games with mentally retarded adults. *American Journal of Occupational Therapy, 35,* 375-382.

King, L. (1978). Toward a science of adaptive responses. *American Journal of Occupational Therapy, 32,* 429-437.

Levine, B. (1979). *Group psychotherapy: Practice and development.* Englewood Cliffs, New Jersey: Prentice-Hall, Inc.

Liberman, R., King, L., DeRisi, W., & McCann, M. (1975). *Personal effectiveness.* Champlain, Illinois: Research Press.

Love, H. (1982). The social skills game. Unpublished therapy game.

Mead, G. (1934). *Mind, self and society.* Chicago: University of Chicago Press.

Meyer, A. (1922). The philosophy of occupational therapy. *Archives of Occupational Therapy, 1,* 1-10.

Mosey, A. (1973). *Activities therapy.* New York: Raven Press.

Mosey, A. (1981). *Occupational therapy: Configuration of a profession.* New York: Raven Press.

Mumford, M. (1974). A comparison of interpersonal skills in verbal and activity groups. *American Journal of Occupational Therapy, 28,* 281-283.

Nochajski, S., & Gordon, C. (1987). The use of Trivial Pursuit in teaching community living skills to adults with developmental disabilities. *American Journal of Occupational Therapy, 41,* 10-15.

Otto, W. (1979). *Play and education: The basic tool for early childhood learning.* Springfield, Illinois: Charles C Thomas.

Raymond, B. (1963). Bridge anyone? *Mental Hospitals, 14,* 226.

Reilly, M. (Ed.) (1974). *Play as exploratory learning.* Beverly Hills: Sage Publications.

Robinson, A. (1977). Play: The arena for the acquisition of rules for competent behavior. *American Journal of Occupational Therapy, 31,* 248-253.

Schwartzberg, S., Howe, M., & McDermott, A. (1982). A comparison of three treatment group formats for facilitating social interaction. *Occupational Therapy in Mental Health: A Journal of Psychosocial Practice and Research, 2,* 1-16.

Takata, N. (1971). The play milieu: A preliminary appraisal. *American Journal of Occupational Therapy, 25,* 281-284.

Vandenberg, B., & Kielhofner, G. (1982). Play in evolution, culture and adaptation. *American Journal of Occupational Therapy, 36,* 20-28.

White, R. (1971). The urge toward competence. *American Journal of Occupational Therapy, 25,* 272-274.

The Effect of a Mime Group on Chronic Adult Psychiatric Clients' Body-Image, Self-Esteem, and Movement-Concept

Deborah L. Probst, MA, OTR
Margot C. Howe, EdD, OTR

SUMMARY. A conceptual model of mime, as a therapeutic group activity, was designed for this study. This model was based on May's (1958) description of three modes of world which characterize the existence of an individual. Eighteen chronic, adult psychiatric clients of a community-based day program met selection criteria for this study. Small mime groups were conducted by the researcher and pre- and post-testing was administered by the facility's staff occupational therapist. Assessment tools consisted of the human figure drawing, the Rosenberg Self-Esteem Scale and a movement-concept scale. Inter-rater reliability between the two raters of the Goodenough rating scale were established for major body parts (.99, $p \leq .05$) and for body proportions (.93, $p \leq .05$). Results of matched pair t-tests (gain score analysis technique) indicated that only body-image as reflected by human figure drawings in regard to proportionality was found to be significantly influenced by mime.

Deborah L. Probst is Occupational Therapist for the Department of Mental Health, Cape Cod and Islands Mental Health and Retardation Center, formerly a graduate student at Tufts University, Medford, MA. This research project was in partial fulfillment of that degree.

Margot C. Howe is Professor, Boston School of Occupational Therapy, Tufts University, Medford, MA 02154.

Appreciation to Laurie York, OTR, for administering the pre-and post-testing, and to the clients of the day program. Appreciation also to the two trained raters. Special thanks to Francis Chamberlain, for teaching the art and discipline of mime.

Address correspondence to: D. L. Probst, OTR, Cape Cod and Islands Mental Health and Mental Retardation Center, County Road, Pocasst, MA 02559.

Qualitative data related to structural and graphic characteristics revealed changes from pre- to post-figure drawings. Clinical observations made during the mime groups were noted. The significant finding of this investigation suggests the potential benefit of mime as a therapeutic activity.

Chronic psychiatric clients frequently experience fundamental problems in relating to themselves, to others, and to their environment. These problems may be interrelated and exhibited by the individual's body-image, self-esteem, and movement. Dissociation of thought, affect, and action may occur when physical actions are limited (Kielhofner, 1983) or when interactions with others are faulty (Schilder, 1950). As Lowen (1967) noted, "When a person loses touch with his body, reality fades out" (p. 6).

The trend in psychiatric treatment is to utilize short-term hospitalization (Loth, 1984) with heavy reliance on psychotropic medication to facilitate release to community programs. However, schizophrenics, as identified by King (1974) often do not respond to medication. Posthuma (1983) in her interview with King, noted King to recommend a neurophysiological approach to treatment,

> In psychiatry we manipulate the nervous system all the time through drugs and I think it is becoming more and more accepted that there are other ways of manipulating the nervous system without drugs. Every time we use muscles, every time we do anything physical, we are changing the design of chemistry of the whole system. (p. 3)

The value of purposeful group activity is well-documented in occupational therapy literature (Fidler & Fidler, 1978; Fine, 1983; Howe & Schwartzberg, 1986; King, 1974; Mosey, 1974). Historically, occupational therapists have viewed activity, including group activity, as a potent healing force (Clark, 1979; Fidler, 1981; Howe & Schwartzberg, 1986; Kielhofner, 1983; Reilly, 1962). In occupational therapy, activity, or occupation, is used to offer individuals opportunities to strengthen their capacities in meeting their needs and responsibilities, in relating to others, and in adapting to the environment. The value of meaningful, purposeful activity underlies diverse theoretical emphases (Fine, 1983; King, 1978; Mosey,

1981). In this study of a mime group, a model of activity is examined within an existential context.

A conceptual model of mime, as a therapeutic group activity in occupational therapy, was designed for a study involving psychiatric clients (Probst, 1987). This design was based on an existential description of three modes of world which characterize the existence of an individual. May (1958) interpreted these three interrelated and simultaneous aspects of world as follows:

> First, there is *Umwelt*, literally meaning "world around"; this is the biological world, generally called in our day the environment. There is, second, the *Mitwelt*, literally the "with world," the world of one's fellow men. The third is *Eigenwelt*, the "own world," the world of relationship to oneself. (p. 61)

Nietzsche (1927) wrote, "one may indeed lie with the mouth, but with the accompanying grimace one nevertheless tells the truth" (p. 469). This study proposes that mime is an instantaneous encounter that is based on self awareness (*Eigenwelt*), resonance with another person (*Mitwelt*), and real involvement with and adaptation to the environment (*Umwelt*). The situations presented within a mime group session take meaning from the clients' experience and immediate situation. Emphasis is on the present; including specific body awareness, relationships within the group, and actions on and responses to (imaginary objects in) the environment. Attention is goal-directed and the activity demands full presence. The aim of the group is for the members to experience, through mime, their body potential, capacity to relate to others, use of objects, and adaptation to environmental situations. The process is active and involves choice.

In the conceptual model (Figure 1), mime is integrally related to the three modes of world. In turn, mime may influence certain concepts that seem to fall within the overlapping areas; that is, body-image, self-esteem, and movement-concept.

Body-image is conceptualized as being determined bio-psychosocially (Schilder, 1942, 1950) and uniquely present as "me" and "me-in-relation-to-others" and to the environment. The adult psychiatric clients in this study show body-image distortions that appear related to their neurological make-ups, physical experiences,

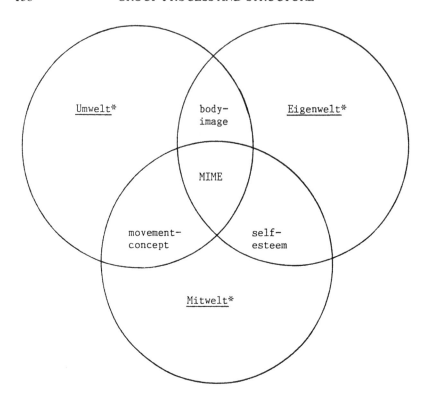

* May (1958) described three modes of world.

Figure 1

Conceptual Model of Mime

relations to others, and environmental conditions and situations. As a group activity, mime is suggested as therapeutic in emphasizing body parts, how big they are, and how they relate to each other (King, 1974; Fowler, King & Snow, 1984), interactions with other group members (Howe & Schwartzberg, 1986), and by adapting to environmental situations, for example, by practicing characterizations (Fleshman & Fryrear, 1981; Lawsen, 1957).

Self-esteem is viewed as arising from a person's relation or bond with the *Eigenwelt, Mitwelt,* and *Umwelt.* The clients who form the population for this study appear to have a weak bonding with self which may denote a lack of self-esteem. This diminished self-esteem seems to underlie esteem for other humans and adjustment to the world. Mime is suggested as a medium through which clients may strengthen a bonding between self-others-environment. For example, when imitating group members, each mime-person is required to match his or her actions with anothers, and in turn, his or her actions are matched by others. This active and decisive process may reinforce the bond motorically and emotionally (Bainbridge et al., 1952; Bruford, 1966; Houle & Wilboux, 1982).

The concept of movement appears intimately connected with *Umwelt,* the world of natural law and natural cycles, the world of biological determination (May, 1983). The idea that "I move myself" is viewed both physically and existentially (Erikson, 1968; Kierkegaard, 1954; Straus, 1958). Kierkegaard (1954) observed, "To become is a movement from the spot, but to become oneself is a movement at the spot" (p. 169). Movement is also profoundly connected with the social world throughout the lifespan (Cratty, 1967; Pitcher & Schultz, 1983). In this study, movement-concept is seen as arising from neurological processes, influenced by primary relationships with others and later peer relations, and becoming incorporated into one's sense of self (Cratty, 1967; Doudlah, 1961; Howe, 1973). Mime may enhance movement-concept by strengthening motor understanding of and confidence in manipulating objects. Nietzsche (1927) recommended, "Remain seated as little as possible; trust no thought that is not born in the open, to the accompaniment of the free bodily motion — nor in which your very muscles do not celebrate a feast" (pp. 836-837).

METHOD

Research Questions

The specific research questions addressed by this study are:

1. What effect does mime, as a therapeutic group activity, have on chronic, adult psychiatric clients' body-image as reflected by their human figure drawings?

2. What effect does mime, as a therapeutic group activity, have on chronic, adult psychiatric clients' self-esteem as reflected by their responses to the Rosenberg Self-Esteem Scale?
3. What effect does mime, as a therapeutic group activity, have on chronic, adult psychiatric clients' movement-concept as reflected by their responses to a movement-concept scale?

Setting

The setting used for this study was a state-contracted, community-based day program in Massachusetts. The program consisted of approximately 35 clients plus an associated drop-in center.

Subjects

The subjects were selected on the basis of the following criteria: they were adults diagnosed according to DSM III Classification, Axes I and II categories including schizophrenic disorder, affective disorder, and personality disorder. Clients with mixed diagnoses were accepted. Diagnoses were verified by the staff occupational therapist as in accordance with DSM III and concordant psychological test results. Clients had to participate in the entire 3-day series of mime groups to be included in the study. Twenty-two clients volunteered for the study and a total of eighteen subjects met selection criteria (Tables 1, 2). Clients who did not volunteer for the study included: those who were new in the program and apparently unwilling to work with an unfamiliar therapist; clients who chose to attend the regular, scheduled Recovery (morning) group held at the same time; those clients who, upon interview, were unable to commit themselves to the subject requirements; those who declined the opportunity with no specific reason except "No, Thank You"; and those clients who typically did not volunteer for, or typically attend groups or activities.

Instruments

Human Figure Drawing. Human figure drawings were used to measure Ss' body-image. The rating scale used for this study was a modified version of the scale developed by Goodenough (1926). This rating scale was constructed as an objective checklist for deter-

TABLE 1

DESCRIPTIVE INFORMATION OF SUBJECTS

BY SEX AND AGE

All Subjects/Sex	Age Mean	Age Range
Female (n = 9)	34.1 years	24-58 years
Male (n = 9)	31.3 years	24-38 years

mining the content, proportional relationships, and structural-graphic characteristics of the drawings.

The list of body parts compiled by Goodenough (1926) was used as a basic list for this modified scale. Results of a pilot test (Simels, 1985) were used to further modify the scale. On this scale, body parts are first noted as being Present or Absent. Second, body parts are examined to determine if they are In Proportion. In the third section, the drawings are analyzed in terms of the following structural-graphic characteristics: type of figure and size and page placement.

The design of this study called for two persons to rate the Ss' human figure drawings. The two raters had been trained by the researcher for a pilot project (Simels, 1985). The inter-rater correlation coefficient for ratings of major body parts was .99 (p ≤ .05). The inter-rater correlation coefficient for ratings of body proportion was .93 (p ≤ .05).

Rosenberg Self-Esteem (RSE) Scale. In this study, the Guttman scoring method employed by Rosenberg (1965) for his ten-item scale was not used. Instead, the four-point scoring method devised by Howe (1973) was chosen as appropriate for this study. Possible scores ranged from a high of 40 points to a low of 10 points.

Movement-Concept (MC) Scale. The instrument used to measure movement-concept was a twenty-item Likert-type rating scale adapted and constructed by Howe (1973). This instrument was de-

TABLE 2

DESCRIPTIVE INFORMATION OF SUBJECTS

BY DIAGNOSES

All Subjects/	Female	Male	Total
Diagnoses, Axis I			
Schizophrenic Disorder			11
Chronic	6	3	
Chronic, Paranoid		2	
Psychotic Disorder			2
Schizoaffective		2	
Affective Disorder			2
Bipolar, Mixed Psychotic		1	
Dysthymic	1		
Anxiety Disorder		1	1
Impulse Disorder	1		1
Organic Brain Syndrome	1		1
Mixed Diagnoses, Axis I			
Substance Abuse	1		1
Mild Mental Retardation	1	1	2
Mixed Diagnoses, Axis II			
Personality Disorder			8
Schizoid	1		
Borderline	1		
Avoidant		1	
Dependent	1	1	
Atypical	2	1	

*Individuals have more than one diagnosis as per DSM III.

signed specifically for adult subjects. Possible scores ranged from a high score of 80 to a low score of 20.

Procedure

The researcher introduced the 3-day mime group program to the clients of the day program and to the clients involved in the associated drop-in center during a pre-scheduled, announced community meeting. The introduction included an invitation to join a mime study, a brief demonstration of mime, an explanation of the time requirements, a description of the pre- and post-testing as paper-pencil activities, and an explanation of the written consent forms.

The staff occupational therapist, familiar with the clients, administered the pre- and post-testing in small groups. Each small group was composed of those clients who were to be in the 3-day mime series scheduled for the following week. The pre-testing was administered approximately one week prior to the mime program. The post-testing was administered immediately following the last mime group of the 3-day series.

The staff occupational therapist administered the human figure drawing first. Standard-size paper and pencils were used. The verbal directions were, "Make a person, a whole person. Draw yourself." Next, the Ss were given the paper-pencil questionnaire that contained the RSE Scale and MC Scale. The staff occupational therapist paced the testing by reading aloud directions for each instrument and assuring completion of all items before proceeding to the following instrument.

The mime program was held on three consecutive days of the week, Tuesday to Thursday mornings from 9-9:45. The groups were conducted in a large (30' by 15'), private room that served as a kitchen/dining and activity room. On completion of the last group (of each mime group series), the staff occupational therapist joined the mime Ss and administered the post-testing. Identical directions for the paper-pencil activities were given. When testing was completed, the researcher invited members of each group series to participate in a final performance to be presented to the day program community. This performance was scheduled for presentation on completion of the mime study.

Description of the Mime Program

The mime groups were designed within an existential context that focused on intensified body awareness, awareness of the movements of others, and awareness, through symbolic visualization, of the environment. Emphasis was placed on the "here and now" shared experience that accentuates genuine human contact. Also considered were the specific sensory integrative capacities facilitated.

Each mime group was based on a consistent format that included: warm-up exercises, opening circle, technique exercises, performance activities, and closing circle. A full description of the mime program is too lengthy to replicate here; however, each section is described briefly to illustrate the important concepts and to capture a visual image of the process.

Warm-up exercises (approximately 15-20 minutes) were done standing in a circle formation. The leader verbally described and demonstrated specific active range of motion (AROM) exercises, balance shifts, and isolations of body parts. The exercises were done in a toe-head progression. Lower extremity exercises began with active stretching, balance shifts, and deep, rhythmical pressure. Several examples of verbatim directions follow:

"Pretend you are walking in an expensive restaurant, and Whoops, you just stepped on a piece of gum! Try to get the gum off."

"Find your balance on one leg; imagine a pole supporting your spine and focus on one point with your eyes (hip is flexed and slightly abducted, knee is flexed). Bend (flex) and point (extend) your raised foot 10 times ($\times$), roll (rotate) to inside (medial) 10$\times$, to outside (lateral) 10$\times$, Repeat with other leg."

"Okay, pretend there is a hook attached to the top of your knee. Slip a chain into the hook and hoist up your knee so the chain is holding your knee up. Your lower leg is dangling free. Swing it in and out 10$\times$. Now, slowly lower the chain and hook up your other knee. Repeat with other leg."

The following warm-up exercises for the waist and ribcage appeared particularly effective in linking motion and emotion:

> "Pretend I'm attaching some yarn here (to leader's sternum) and I'm pulling it. Watch this movement. Here (to S), you pull the yarn for me. My shoulders don't move, my ribcage does. Practice."
>
> "Now point your finger to your chest, and let it collapse in, just a little. Feel that, what is that emotion? And use your yarn to pull your chest out. What is that emotion?"

Upper extremity exercises emphasized freedom of movement and then focused on purposeful movement, for example, rolls, swings, then,

> "Reach way forward and grab some . . . money, pull it in, reach again . . . in all directions. Fill up your pockets!"
>
> "Shake your hands, real hard, now flap them, now shake them."

Lastly, neck and facial exercises included slow, bilateral neck rolls, scalp massage, and facial expressions, "With no one seeing, make some faces, tighten up and frown, look mean, open up and stretch your face, and smile."

The *opening circle* consisted of imitation of group members. The leader initiated imitation by visually focusing on the S opposite, putting finger to mouth to indicate silence, and imitating (mirror image) each action and facial expression made. Verbally, the leader stage whispered that everyone was to copy that person until he or she *froze* and pointed to the next person to be imitated. Each person took a turn around the circle. This section was approximately 5 minutes.

In the opening circle, the leader's actions consisted of: on first day, "scratching an itch"; on second day, "looking in a mirror and preening"; and on last day, "miming walking on a hot day, buying and eating a dripping ice cream cone."

The next section consisted of teaching *mime technique* (Chamberlain, personal communication, 1983-1984; Lawsen, 1957; Sayre, 1959; Shepard, 1971; Stolzenberg, 1979; Walker, 1969).

Each group in the 3-day program focused on specific techniques. This section was approximately 10-15 minutes.

On the first day, techniques involved manipulation of objects: rope pulling and tug-of-war; pushing furniture; and mopping the floor. This action was primarily non-verbal, except for transitions, clarifications, and jokes. Emphasis was placed on pushing hard, using tonic muscle groups, and heavy work patterns.

On the second day of the mime program, technique exercises focused on expression of motion and expression of emotion. The Ss were instructed to move across the floor in a manner that would show sneakiness, shyness, anger, sadness, determination, and anticipation. Expression of an emotional change was suggested, specifically, "Move as if . . . your best friend had failed an important test . . . now show that your friend took it again, was waiting to hear, waiting (all nervous) . . . and passed!"

On the third day of the mime program, technique exercises focused on characterization. Animal characters were acted out first. The leader demonstrated a "bird" with gliding movements. The Ss were instructed to mime a cat playing and scratching. Next, the Ss were asked to "become humans with animal-like characteristics." The leader demonstrated a woman walking with a gliding gait stroking her hair. She asked the Ss to mime a man eating a hamburger. Lastly, the Ss were invited to mime a teenager walking and smoking a cigarette and an adult hurrying (these were done as a group, with members randomly walking around the room).

The next section consisted of brief *mime performances* by each of the group members. Each S chose one of the techniques taught on the respective day: sketches involving manipulation of objects; expression of motion and emotion; and telling a story with characterization. In setting the stage for performance, the leader invited the Ss to sit on chairs on one side of the floor space. She emphasized the importance of attention to the present, economy of movement, and focus on silently portraying where?, who?, what?, and why? (intent) in the performance of mime. In this section, the leader was part of the "audience" and offered some verbal critiques of technique, not content.

The *closing circle* of the group consisted of brief imitation of movement. The leader asked the Ss to re-form a circle. Directions for the opening were repeated, but mimes were limited to imitation of one action per S.

In the closing circle, the leader's actions included: "dribbling a basketball and taking a measured shot"; "assuming a slumped posture and taking a drag on a cigarette"; and on the last day, "bowing in Thank you to each group member."

RESULTS

In total, eighteen subjects completed the 3-day mime program. Only the influence of mime on body-image, as reflected by Ss' human figure drawings in regard to proportionality, was found to be significant using the Students t-test of pre and post scores. Findings indicated no significant differences in body-image as reflected by Ss' human figure drawings in regard to major body parts, responses to the RSE Scale, nor responses to the MC Scale (Table 3). As indicated in Table 3, one S refused the human figure drawing, writing, "I can't do this" on her paper. A different S refused the RSE Scale with the explanation, "I can't answer these questions." As Ss fulfilled the primary criteria of participating in the entire 3-day series of mime groups, they were included in the results of the study.

Certain qualitative data pertaining to Ss' human figure drawings provided descriptive information related to the structural and graphic characteristics. Changes from pre- to post-drawings were noted in regard to type of figure drawn, height of figure, and space organization.

The Ss' human figure drawings were examined by the two trained raters to determine type of figure drawn. Seventeen matched pairs of figures were reviewed and the raters found that: in the pre-drawings, Ss drew 3 stick figures, 2 profiles, and 12 full face, body front figures; in the post-drawings, Ss drew 2 stick figures and 15 full face, body front figures.

Although the height of the figure drawings differed minimally from pre- to post-testing (pre-drawing, $\bar{\bar{x}} = 6.0$; post-drawing, $\bar{\bar{x}} = 5.8$), there was notable variability in drawing size from subject to subject and from picture to picture. Figure height from subject to subject ranged from 1-1/2" to 10-1/2". Size variability of matched pairs of drawings ranged from no difference to seven inches differ-

TABLE 3

RESULTS OF MATCHED PAIR T-TEST FOR SUBJECTS' SCORES,

FIGURE DRAWINGS, RSE SCALE, AND MOVEMENT-CONCEPT SCALE

	Pre-test[a]	Post-test	Subject T-Scores
Figure Drawings	n = 17	n = 17	
Major Body Parts	x = 10.97	x = 11.76	ts = 1.23 (df = 16)
	sd = 3.18	sd = 3.68	
Body Proportion	x = 3.79	x = 6.53	ts = 5.48* (df = 16)
	sd = 2.15	sd = 2.49	
RSE Scale	n = 17	n = 17	
	x = 25.5	x = 26.6	ts = 1.23 (df = 16)
	sd = 6.32	sd = 4.81	
Movement-Concept Scale	n = 18	n = 18	
	x = 56.33	x = 55.66	ts = -.27 (df = 17)
	sd = 8.34	sd = 9.20	

[a] One S refused the HFD pre-test and one S refused the RSE Scale pre-test

* significant at p<.05.

ence. No pattern of change was discerned; that is, figures were drawn both bigger and smaller in post-testing.

Of interest was the page placement of Ss' human figure drawings. All figures, except one pre-drawing, were placed left of center or in the center of the page. In the pre-drawings, 11 Ss drew figures left of center, 5 drew figures in the center, and one S drew a figure right of center; in the post-drawings, 6 Ss drew figures left of center and 11 Ss drew figures in the center of the page.

Structural and graphic changes revealed in Ss' drawings but not detected by the rating scale included: posture of figure, position of body parts, joint attachments, clothing, and style/technique. Two striking examples of figure drawing changes apparent on observation but not reflected by statistic scores nor description were (a) pre-drawing figure drawn in rigid stance with unfocused eyes (eye sockets not closed, eye direction ambiguous) and post-drawing figure drawn jumping rope with focused, directed eye gaze and (b) pre-drawing drawn with full facial features but stick figure body with no hands or feet and post-drawing drawn with no facial features but complete body outline in pose of dynamic movement.

Clinical observations made during the mime groups were not included in the assessment tools used in this study. The clients who participated in the study were (a) on time, (b) attentive to the researcher and to each other, and (c) clearly enjoying the groups. Intensified attention was demonstrated by task-appropriate eye contact, accurate mirroring including subtle adjustments during the imitation sections of the mime groups, and ability to concentrate on and demonstrate understanding of mime techniques. Enjoyment of the mime groups was demonstrated by laughter and positive comments made during and after the mime groups. Approximately half of the subjects involved in the study volunteered to be in a Halloween mime performance for the entire day program. This behavior was not typical for this group of chronic, adult clients.

Limitations

Certain limitations of this study need to be acknowledged. While an attempt was made to use objective data collection methods, the sample size was small, not randomly selected, and there was no way to control for possible Hawthorne effect bias. Therefore, results of the study cannot claim to represent any other population.

In terms of the activity used, this study was limited by client receptivity to mime; that is, to what extent the clients were willing to be engaged in the activity and with the leader of the activity.

This study was also limited to the degree to which the measurement tools actually represent the variables being analyzed, and the appropriateness of the measurement tools for the population included.

CONCLUSION AND IMPLICATIONS

Implications for Using Mime as a Therapeutic Activity and Recommendations for Future Research

The findings of this study indicate that it is possible, by means of designing a model of an activity, to systematically investigate a specific treatment modality. A conceptual model, such as the design used for mime, could be constructed for other activities used in occupational therapy.

Results of this study support that a mime group could be used to effect chronic, adult psychiatric clients' body-image. For example, mime could be used to explore body awareness if a client's human figure drawing reflected problems with proportionality. Further research appears indicated as to the meaning of chronic, adult psychiatric clients' human figure drawings in regard to proportionality.

Not measured here, but of potential benefit are also the effect of mime on body movement and the effect of mime on verbal communication. An intriguing observation in this investigation was that certain clients clearly found mime meaningful as noted by their punctuality, intensified attention, and enjoyment. Perhaps this observation might be based on the ability of these clients, through mime, to express themselves and to communicate on a non-verbal, person-to-person level (in an existential sense, May, 1983). Further research utilizing video equipment might capture clinical changes not detected by paper-pencil assessment tools.

It seems important to refine this study. As noted, the study was the initial design of a conceptual model of mime, and the first time that the effect of mime on the interrelating variables of body-image, self-esteem, and movement-concept was explored. Further exploration of client receptivity to mime due to diagnoses and prior group and physical experiences might clarify questions relating to treatment effectiveness. It seems warranted that a larger sample of clients could establish more predictive patterns.

In respect to the variables studied, the effect of mime on each of them might be explored. Thus, each concept could be examined more fully, including modifications of the instruments used.

Specifically in terms of the instruments used, another recommendation is to refine the rating scale with the client population involved. A refinement of this study should modify the human figure drawing rating scale to include a greater range of options for major body parts present, more specific proportionality comparisons, and a greater range of options for structural and graphic characteristics. The instruments used to assess self-esteem and movement-concept should be validated in regard to the population involved. Adding the NOSIE-30 as an outcome measure might further clarify behavioral change.

A final recommendation is that a study be conducted to assess the effect of a mime group when used for longer periods of time. This study was devised as a 3-day series as a preliminary investigation. Research investigating the neurological and physical processes inherent in mime as a movement-oriented activity would necessitate longer-term client involvement.

REFERENCES

American Psychiatric Association. (1980). *Diagnostic and statistical manual of mental disorders.* (3rd. ed.). Washington, DC: Author.

Bainbridge, G., Duddington, A.E., Collingdon, M., & Gardner, C.E. (1952). Dance-mime: A contribution to treatment in psychiatry. *Journal of Mental Science, 99* 308-314.

Clark, P. N. (1979). Human development through occupation: A philosophy and conceptual model for practice, part 2. *American Journal of Occupational Therapy, 33* (9), 577-585.

Cratty, B. J. (1967). *Social dimensions of physical activity.* Englewood Cliffs, NJ: Prentice Hall.

Doudlah, A.M. (1961). *The relationship between the self-concept, the body-image and the movement-concept of college freshmen women with low and average motor ability.* Unpublished thesis, University of North Carolina.

Erikson, E.H. (1968). *Identity, youth and crisis.* New York: W.W. Norton.

Fidler, G. (1981). From crafts to competence. *American Journal of Occupational Therapy, 35* (9), 567-580.

Fidler, G.S. & Fidler, J.W. (1978, May-June). Doing and becoming: Purposeful action and self-actualization. *American Journal of Occupational Therapy, 32* (5),305-310.

Fine, S. (1983), Occupational therapy: The role of rehabilitation and purposeful activity in mental health practice. *American Occupational Therapy Association Monograph.*

Fleshman, B. & Fryrear, J. L. (1981). *The arts in therapy.* Chicago: Nelson-Hall.

Fowler, R. H., King, L. J., & Snow, B. A. (1984). The use of dance in therapy. *Sensory Integration Special Interest Section Newsletter, 7* (2), 2-3.

Goodenough, F. L. (1926). *Measurement of intelligence by drawings.* Chicago: World Books.

Houle, B. & Wilboux, S. (1982). New mime in North America, San Francisco, CA. In T. Leabhart (Ed.). (1980, 1981, 1982). *Mime Journal.* Claremont, CA: Pamona College Theatre.

Howe, M. C. (1973). *A comparison of the self-esteem, body-image, and movement-concept of adults in different age groups.* Unpublished doctoral dissertation, Boston University, Department of Education.

Howe, M. C. & Schwartzberg, S. L. (1986). *A functional approach to groupwork in occupational therapy.* Philadelphia: J. B. Lippincott.

Kielhofner, G. (1983). *Health through occupation: Theory and practice in occupational therapy.* Philadelphia: F.A. Davis.

Kierkegaard, S. (transl. by W. Lowrie, 1954). *Fear and trembling and the sickness unto death.* Princeton, NJ: Princeton University Press.

King, L. J. (1974). A sensory integrative approach to schizophrenia. *American Journal of Occupational Therapy, 28* (9), 529-536.

King, L. J. (1978). Occupational therapy research in psychiatry: A perspective, *American Journal of Occupational Therapy, 32* (1), 15-18.

King, L. J. (1983). Occupational therapy and neuropsychiatry. *Occupational Therapy in Mental Health, 3* (1), 1-13.

Lawsen, J. (1957). *Mime: The theory and practice of expressive gesture with a description of historical development.* London: Pitman.

Loth, R. (1984, July). After the Beverly fire: Another look at patient-release policy. *Boston Phoenix,* pp. 1, 8-9, 32, 34-35.

Lowen, A. (1967). *The betrayal of the body.* New York: Collier MacMillan.

May, R. (1983). *The discovery of being: Writings in existential psychology.* New York: W. W. Norton.

May, R., Angel, E., & Ellenberger, H.F. (Eds.). (1958). *Existence: A new dimension in psychiatry and psychology.* New York: Basic Books.

Mosey, A. C. (1973). *Activities Therapy.* New York: Raven Press.

Mosey, A. C. (1981). *Occupational therapy: Configuration of a profession.* New York: Raven Press.

Nietzsche, F. (1927). *The philosophy of Nietzsche.* New York: The Modern Library.

Pitcher, E. G. & Schultz, L.H. (1983). *Boys and girls at play: The development of sex roles.* New York: Praeger.

Posthuma, B. W. (1983). Sensory integration in mental health: Dialogue with Lorna Jean King. *Occupational Therapy in Mental Health, 3* (4), 1-9.

Reilly, M. (1962). 1961 Eleanor Clark Slagle Lecture: Occupational therapy can be one of the great ideas of 20th century medicine. *American Journal of Occupational Therapy, 16* (1), 1-9.

Rosenberg, M. (1965). *Society and the adolescent self-image.* Princeton, NJ: Princeton University Press.

Sayre, G. (1959). *Creative miming.* London: Herbert Jenkins.

Schilder, P. (1942). *Mind: Perception and thought in their constructive aspects.* New York: Columbia University Press.

Schilder, P. (1950). *The image and appearance of the human body: Studies in the constructive energies of the psyche.* New York: McGraw-Hill.

Shepard, R. (1971). *Mime: The technique of silence.* New York: Drama Book Specialists.

Simels, D. L. (1985). *The effect of mime on the body-image of schizophrenic and other psychiatric clients.* Unpublished manuscript. Tufts University, Boston School of Occupational Therapy, Medford.

Stolzenberg, M. (1979). *Exploring mime.* New York: Sterling.

Straus, E. W. (1958). Aesthesiology and hallucinations. In R. May, E. Angel & H.F. Ellenberger (Eds.). (1958). *Existence: A new dimension in psychiatry and psychology.* New York. Basic Books.

Walker, K. S. (1969). *Eyes on mime: Language without speech.* New York: John Day.

Using Robots in a Group
with the Neuropsychologically Impaired:
Achieving a Sense of Control
Over the Environment

Valnère P. McLean, MS, OTR/L, FAOTA

SUMMARY. Having a sense of control over one's environment can be achieved in a group of neuropsychologically-impaired patients through the use of robots. Having a sense of control can help restore good feelings about oneself. The rationale for developing such a group is discussed. The structure and process of the group are illustrated in a description of a typical group session.

Having administered an occupational therapy assessment to five patients on a neuropsychological ward, I was impressed by the mixture of functional abilities and functional deficits of these patients. I realized that although these patients were dependent in self care and safety, they did have some functionally productive and adaptive behaviors which were being ignored. The patients seemed trapped, defenseless and suffering. They needed stimulation.

In humanistic thinking, the belief is that man can assume responsibility for himself and has the ability to understand his own limitations and potential. His reason for being is shaped by his own perceptions of his world. Therefore, although neurological and emotional

Valnère P. McLean is a self-employed occupational therapist. She provides contracted services and consultation services to home health agencies, extended care facilities and in-patient psychiatric hospitals. She is part-time faculty at Quinnipiac College, Hamden, CT. Mailing address: 110 Gunger Hill Road, Higganum, CT 06441.

155

trauma have modified these patients' abilities, couldn't they be "acting" people instead of always being "acted upon"?

Several theoretical assumptions contributed to forming the type of group these patients seemed to need.

White (1959) explains that one can explore the environment if one does not experience fear. To promote an effect, one needs to experience a competent interaction with the environment. Perceptual motor skills, cognitive skills and adaptive mechanisms build toward competence, achievement and an effective interaction with the environment.

Rogers claims that clients seek help because of a feeling of "basic helplessness, powerlessness and inability to make decisions or effectively direct their own lives" (Corey, 1986, p. 106). In therapy, they learn and experience their own responsibility in making changes and controlling what happens (Rogers, 1961).

Maslow's (1968) theories of self actualization emphasize the value of satisfying needs, and the experiencing of a sense of achievement and a "healthy self-esteem and self confidence." "The person who hasn't conquered, withstood and overcome continues to feel doubtful that he *could*" (p. 4).

Goldstein developed his theories of self-actualization while studying brain-injured soldiers. He believes that a person has to come to terms with his environment. The environment provides the opportunities for self-actualization or it hampers these opportunities through lack of objects or the presence of impeding conditions. Self-actualization and mastery over the environment come from within a person (Hall and Lindzey, 1978).

These patients needed to take responsibility. They needed an opportunity to assert control over their environment. If this is to be achieved in a group format, what format would succeed? What structure should the group assume? And what activities would provide opportunities for these patients to experience control?

When Howe and Schwartzberg (1986) published their work "A Functional Approach to Group Work in Occupational Therapy," the model verified the idea for a patient group. Being reassured that a group could be managed even when it did not have a unified goal or interdependent task, a patient group was started. The strengths and limitations of these patients seemed well able to fit into a "collective'' group format. Moreover, this group of patients did have a unified goal, i.e., achieving a sense of control over the environment, although the interdependent task work done in the group would be limited.

THE STRUCTURE OF THE GROUP

"The way in which a group is structured will greatly affect patients' ability to achieve improved social skills" (Morse [Ed.], 1986, p. 136). The authors discuss the applicability of Mosey's (1986) framework of group levels to brain-injured patients. Perhaps these patients could function at the project group level. Using the therapist as the group leader and given a simple task, each patient could assume responsibility for a portion of the task and contribute to its accomplishment. Each group session needed to be a single entity and would follow the five-stage group process developed by Ross and Burdick (1981). Thus, the demands on each patient and the process of the group would be predictable and organized.

Finally, we had the rationale for the group, and its structure and process selected. We needed an activity—an activity that would provide the patients with a sense of control. An idea came to the author after observing her three-year-old niece, Vivian, play with a robot. At first she was afraid of it as it moved about. But, when she was given the remote control unit, Vivian discovered that she was controlling the robot. Her behavior changed from being fearful and petulant to gleeful and positive. Obviously, a sense of control over the environment could be achieved through robots, programmable robots and remote controlled robots, those that respond to voice commands and those that are operated mechanically. Thus, an activity was found. Five robots were chosen: Omnibot, Verbot, Armatron robot arm, a small spaceship-like robot called Movit and another small robot similar to Omnibot and Verbot to look at, but only having the capabilities of moving forward and backward and carrying something very small. Omnibot is our largest robot. It can record and play tapes, project a person's voice through a built-in speaker, or program into its memory (onto cassette) movements, speeches, dialogues, songs, etc., that can be played back immediately or at a programmed time. Also, Omnibot can transport items on its tray. Verbot is a small voice-operated robot that can follow up to eight functions—five directional functions, two carrying functions and one social function. Armatron has a "jointed" arm that can be rotated, moved in four directions and a pincer "hand" to pick up, move and release objects. This is operated by two joysticks. Movit, the small spaceship-like robot, moves rapidly in any direction and responds with directional changes through clapping, banging or snapping sounds. A sixth robot, that has similar operations to Armatron, but can pour liquids as well, is to be purchased soon.

ACTIVITY ANALYSIS

In order to be sure the robots would be versatile and constructively useful, an activity analysis was done. Four main components were considered: Sensory motor, Cognitive, Social and Adaptability.

Sensory Motor

Posture-positioning: The robots can encourage postural changes and mobility, speed of change, weight shifting and immediate feedback on performance. For example, operating Omnibot to transport an item on his tray requires reaching to place something on the tray, positioning to use the remote control unit, and making postural adjustments as the robot moves to its intended destination.

Visual motor: Visual scanning and head adjustments are required in operating the robots' controls and observing the robots' responses or following their movements. Visual processing (discrimination, gestalt and orientation in space) is needed while selecting the robot's path of movement, assessing the environment for obstacles, locating desired objects and directing the robots to the desired objects, etc. Also, eye/hand coordination is enhanced as operation of each robot is mastered.

Sensory awareness: This can be accomplished kinesthetically, through fine motor operation of the controls, such as the grasp strength and finger pressure needed, and the force required and judgement about the carrying-weight capacity of the robots. Left/

right side awareness can be incorporated into the robot's movements and location of objects.

Cognitive

Orientation and Attention, Organization (following directions, planning), Memory, Problem Solving: The robots' particular value is in providing goal-directed activities, such as carrying a written message to another group member, picking up an item off the table with the pincer hands of one kind of robot, transporting the item, and giving it to someone else, transferring the item to another robot or displaying the item to the whole group. The operator has to decide what he wants to do, plan how he will do it, understand the capacities of the robot, adjust and problem solve difficulties and recall previous experiences from past group sessions.

Tangible/Intangible; Concrete/Abstract; Feedback; Response Time: The activities performed by the robots are tangible in that the robots can either do or not do what the operator wants. The tasks are concrete, there is a beginning and an end to each task, the outcome is obvious, the feedback is immediate and the response time is immediate enough to demonstrate cause and effect, but easily adjustable to the operator's processing needs and capabilities.

Social

Emotional Expression; Intrapersonal/Interpersonal: The importance of dealing with frustration and impulse control can be demonstrated and discussed. The robots will not become frustrated but they can only perform if the correct information is provided. Unacceptable demands do not work.

Robots, by the feedback they give in their immediate responses and through the goal directed activities they can be commanded to perform, provide opportunities for understanding one's own behavior and in demonstrating socially acceptable behaviors towards others, such as waiting one's turn, doing something for someone else and helping another person be successful.

Adaptability

The tasks performed using the robots can be broken down into steps. One patient can do all of the steps or several patients can perform different steps in the one task. Those that have good speech patterns can use the voice controlled robots and those who can perform motorically can use the mechanically operated robots. The robots can be operated from various positions and by different parts of the body. For example, the joy stick can be operated with the heel of the hand or the elbow if the hand is non-functional.

A TYPICAL GROUP

In all, eight patients attend the group. Four are post-traumatic brain-injured, one has Alzheimer's, two have Huntington's chorea, and one, a young woman, sustained a cerebrovascular accident and has an organic brain syndrome. At each group session, two tables are placed side by side in the center of the room and the patients are grouped around them. The tables provide a central focus and a concrete boundary for the group, in addition to making the activities accessible to every group member.

Stage One — Sensory Motor

The group starts with the female patients greeting the male patients. Each patient is encouraged to say the name of the patient he or she is greeting. This is followed by discussion about the day and anything special that needs to be mentioned. One patient (non-verbal) selects a descriptor about the weather from a pile of cards. He gives it to another patient who puts it in the "hand" of the Armatron robot and mechanically rotates it around so that each patient is able to read it, say the description aloud, and comment and elaborate on it. Other variations to this are discussions about a special holiday occurring during that month, memories about the holiday, and ways to enjoy it this month. This leads into exercises.

Stage Two — Movement

Sometimes the therapist is the leader of the exercise activities and sometimes the leader role is shared. Exercises include stretching, reaching and rotating trunk and arms. This portion ends with a fine motor task, such as opening and closing a packet, an envelope, etc., or manipulating an object such as a segmented plastic snake, or controlling the Movit robot.

Stage Three — Perceptual Integration

This stage requires the greatest use of the robots. Activities are structured so that concepts of direction, speed, left/right orientation, use of space, and maintaining spatial boundaries are incorporated.

Stage Four — Cognitive Function

Frequently, stage four blends with stage three. The activities emphasize attention to task, problem-solving and decision-making requirements and memory.

One activity the patients thoroughly enjoy requires the use of Armatron and Verbot or Omnibot, depending on whether the focus needs to be on verbal or motor commands. A "secret" message is sealed in an envelope and given to Verbot or Omnibot. The patient responsible for either Verbot or Omnibot has to transport the message to the patient using the Armatron. The Armatron has to pick up the message and hand it to its operator who can open the envelope and share the message.

The sense of pleasure, accomplishment, success and control felt by all members in the group, including the therapist, is moving. The five stages have provided a logical way to process the group, the robots have responded, rebelled, and rewarded each member as he or she has used them in his or her own specialized way, and, most importantly, each group member has had a moment of being in control.

Stage Five — Termination

Stage five comes naturally with the completion of a successful activity, a refreshment delivered by Omnibot, and expectations for the next group session.

The robot group has been held one time weekly for sixteen and one half months at the time of this writing. It is considered effective in that it has demonstrated the preserved functional abilities of many of the patients participating. The author has been able to use the information gained from observing the functional behavior of these patients to justify the purchase of two computers. Administration agrees that the head-injured patients, in particular, have demonstrated how they have benefited from a predictable, well-structured environment, well-planned and controlled sensory stimulation, and challenging and motivating activities. The patients have shown that they want to ''act'' and be in control. The following case illustrates how one patient has responded.

Ed is a thirty-seven-year-old white male who sustained a traumatic brain injury in a motorcycle accident sixteen years ago. He experienced a loss of consciousness of greater than two months, followed by an undetermined period of amnesia. An EEG record eight years later indicated a severe diffuse slowing and diffuse atrophic changes.

Current problems include left hemiplegia, left below knee amputation, dysphasia, dysarthria, incontinence of urine, left third nerve palsy, exotropia and dislocated lens and behavioral dysfunction characterized by non-compliance.

Pre-traumatically, Ed had difficulty with impulse control. His academic history indicated truancy and antisocial adjustment. He has a history of polysubstance abuse and he had been in jail five times for minor theft and fighting. Reportedly, he was employed as an accountant and he was married.

A review of Ed's post-traumatic test scores and evaluations provide the following information. Ed's strengths are: functionally adequate right hand fine motor speed, auditory attention and verbal comprehension, figure ground perception and spatial orientation. He is capable of simple motor planning and has some preserved capacity for abstraction.

His weaknesses are in his inappropriate social behavior, his visual scanning, visual field and left-side neglect problems, his postural instability and left-side weakness with resultant mobility loss, and his communication difficulties, such as productive speech, reading and writing problems.

His loss of cognitive and intellectual functioning, combined with his physical and communicative limitations, have forced Ed into a frustratingly dependent status. Furthermore, he is forced into even greater isolation by his inappropriate social behavior. On the ward, Ed does none of his self-care activities with the exception of feeding himself. If he were exposed to a simple fine-motor eye/hand coordination activity, could he learn to perform the activity independently? He seemed to be an appropriate candidate for the robot group, and was included in the group with this question in mind.

Operation of a robot would be a new activity for him and would provide opportunities for him to use his strengths and remaining abilities. During the group, Ed used the Armatron robot.

While operating Armatron, Ed could use his stronger auditory verbal comprehension abilities, his simple motor-planning abilities, his cognitive abilities, such as directional concepts, his ability to plan and sequence steps in a simple task, and to remember the operational steps needed. Operation of Armatron also made use of his preserved capacity for abstraction in the simple problem solving that is necessary and the understanding needed to achieve the desired outcome of a completed task.

The areas that could have proven to be a problem were his difficulties in visual scanning and his limited visual field.

Ed was able to attend fifty-one groups over the sixteen and one-half months' period and has had twenty-two opportunities to operate the Armatron robot in the group. He did not see or operate the robot at any other time. At the end of this period, Ed was tested in his abilities to operate the Armatron robot independently. He was taken to a quiet environment and was alone with one observer. Using the pincer hand of the robot, Ed was asked to take a 4 × 6 card with a weather descriptor written on one side and display it to the observer. There was to be no step by step instruction on the operation of the robot or verbal cueing after the initial task instructions were given. The task was expected to take about five minutes to complete.

Ed did the entire task independently and in less time — three minutes and ten seconds. Thus, in a group environment with many distractions and delays, Ed did learn a task and he did demonstrate that he has the ability to conceptualize an outcome and utilize his remaining memory and other cognitive functions to complete this simple task. Also, in all the group sessions Ed attended, his behavior was appropriate. He waited his turn, encouraged other members who were having difficulties, concentrated on the activity at hand, and was cooperative in the shared responsibilities of performing the task. In this group, Ed demonstrated socially appropriate behavior.

CONCLUSION

This article is based on humanistic thinking which states that man can assume responsibility for himself. If man can be action-oriented instead of acted upon he can develop a sense of control. This, in turn, leads to productive behavior and learning. An explanation of a group that provides opportunities for control and a description of a patient who participated in the group serve to illustrate how patients can take responsibility and participate actively. The next step is to take these abilities and include them in the patients' daily routines.

REFERENCES

Corey, G. (1986). *Theory and Practice of Counseling and Psychotherapy* (3rd. ed.). Monterey, California: Brooks/Cole Publishing Company.

Hall, C.S., Lindzey, G. (1978). *Theories of Personality* (3rd. ed.). New York: John Wiley and Sons.

Howe, M.C., Schwartzberg, S.L. (1986). *A Functional Approach to Group Work in Occupational Therapy*. Philadelphia: J. B. Lippincott.

Maslow, A.H. (1968). *Toward a Psychology of Being* (2nd. ed.). New York: Van Nostrand Reinhold.

Guzik, J. (1986). *Brain Injury: Cognitive and Prevocational Approaches to Rehabilitation*. In P.A. Morse (Ed.). New York: Tiresias Press Inc.

Mosey, A.C. (1976). *Activities Therapy*. New York: Raven Press.

Rogers, Carl R. (1961). *On Becoming a Person*. Boston: Houghton Mifflin.

Ross, M., Burdick, D. (1981). *Sensory Integration: A Training Manual for Therapists and Teachers for Regressed, Psychiatric and Geriatric Patient Groups*. New Jersey: Slack Inc.

White, R. (1959). Motivation Reconsidered: The Concept of Competence. *Psychological Review* 66(5): 297-333.